"This book is a reflection on the important things ir _____ appreciate them. It is easy to read, and everyone can rel _____ ....al and sometimes personal stories. This is a 'must read' and a reminder for all of us that we each can live a more balanced and healthy life . . . if we choose to."

—*Terri L. Kane, BSN, MBA, regional vice president, Southwest Region, Intermountain Healthcare, CEO Dixie Regional Medical Center*

"*WholeFIT: Wellness for Life* is one of the best books I have seen in integrating principles of life, health, and fitness as it relates to the general well-being of an individual. The editor's approach of connecting the sociological aspects of life to physiological outcomes is one I feel will greatly benefit the reader. This rare approach provides the reader with useful tools in addressing healthy lifestyle choices that are easy to understand yet will result in healthy outcomes."

—*Richard B. Williams, PhD, president, Dixie State University*

"In an era where the epidemics are not so much infectious agents as diseases of lifestyle, this book is a welcome offering. Utilizing the expertise of a variety of professionals who contribute easy-to-understand advice on everything from motivation, exercise, diet, and relationships, it harkens back to the wellness movement of the 1970s with a new and modern flavor. What Drs. Donald Ardell and John Travis did then to introduce the concept of 'wellness' instead of a focus on illness in that era, DuPree and colleagues bring to us today.

"This book will be a useful guide for individuals seeking life change as well as those such as health coaches, counselors, and other health professionals seeking to facilitate their progress toward wellness and change. The complex interplay of body, mind, spirit, work, relationships, emotion, love, leisure, and community all must be balanced for a fully healthy life plan. The achievement of salutogenesis, the generation of health, as opposed to pathogenesis, the development of disease, is the ultimate goal, and this lovely book offers a roadmap to such a goal."

—*Victor S. Sierpina, MD, ABFM, ABIHM; director, Medical Student Education Program; WD and Laura Nell Nicholson Family Professor of Integrative Medicine; professor, family medicine; University of Texas Medical Branch*

"It's clear beyond reason that true health is more than just diet and exercise. To perform better, align with purpose, and experience contentment, we must capture and activate a collective effort of all energies and resources that surround us on a daily basis. WholeFIT is the method for making this happen. Jared and his colleagues create a principle-centered and wholistic approach to complete wellness, inside and out, in small steps. Get WholeFIT today!"

—*Joe Jacobi, Olympic gold medalist, Whitewater Canoe Slalom, performance coach, professional speaker, network television commentator, and former CEO of USA Canoe/Kayak*

"When I consider all there is to learn and all there is to do in this life, [this book] reminds me of what is truly important. We are all connected. The different areas of our lives are connected. Life fulfillment and peace comes from living our lives in a way that is meaningful to us, considering all the opportunities we have to expand our wellness. *WholeFIT* tells us that true wellness is more than avoiding disease or sickness. Wellness is about all the parts that make us who we are—our relationships, hearts, minds, bodies, spirit, resources, careers, passions, and life purpose. I highly recommend this book for those that want to become better. Not in the stressful, guilt-ridden way of, 'I need to do better.' Rather, this book is a warm invitation, a gentle embrace, a support, and a friend. Whether you are someone looking for better life balance or an employer that wants to help their employees find more happiness and purpose in life, *WholeFIT* is a welcome change of pace and outlook on how to truly be well. Read it—you will love it!"

—*Mary Michelle Scott, PhD, president of Fishbowl, and contributor to* Harvard Business Review *and* Forbes

"The authors offer a theory of living that is informed by research, practice, and thoughtful reflection on the experience of living. These are not experts instructing from the ivory tower. The authors walk alongside the reader, inviting the reader to reflect upon their own process. The careful reader will come to know something about the life choices of the authors, which in my judgment, enhances their credibility. Each chapter offers step-by-step guidance on how to create a new, healthier homeostasis, and encouragement to start *now*."

—*Candyce S. Russell, PhD, professor emerita, marriage and family therapy, Kansas State University*

"*WholeFIT: Wellness for Life* is a must-read that is uniquely and masterfully written by several authors and then integrated and organized into a WholeFIT approach for lifelong wellness. It is rich with ideas and invaluable insights that could have a huge impact on your life. It is a book of knowledge containing recipes for real life success, integrating our minds, our hearts, our bodies, our health, our relationships, and our spirituality. It provides tools that one needs to achieve better health and more passion in day to day living. This is a life-changer must-read book that will help map the journey of wellness for the rest of your life. A book I will share with both my personal and my professional friends."

—*Coleen M. Andruss, MD, Board-Certified Internal Medicine and Bariatrics, owner, Healthy Lifestyles Clinic, Saint George, Utah*

"The road to better health is something that we are all searching for, but we don't always know how to find it. As resource, *WholeFIT: Wellness for Life* provides readers with multiple on-ramps to begin (or continue) their own journey to well-being and happiness. Dr. DuPree and his coauthors do a great job of highlighting the research associated with physical, mental, spiritual, and relational health and making these complex concepts approachable and immediately applicable. Each chapter is motivating because the overall tone is, 'You can make important changes and here is how.' I will recommend this book to my students, my family, and my clients."

—Roy A Bean, PhD, associate professor and program director, marriage and family therapy, School of Family Life, Brigham Young University

"Gone are the days where we compartmentalize health, separating the mind from the body and spirit, the individual from the family, and the family from the community. This book is an excellent compilation of ideas from scholars and mental health professionals who share what they have learned personally and professionally about rebalancing one's life to achieve whole health and wellness. Authors offer personal stories to complement their professional ideas in an easy-to-read resource that you won't want to put down!"

—Jennifer Hodgson, PhD, LMFT: professor and director of the Medical Family Therapy doctoral program at East Carolina University; past president of the Collaborative Family Healthcare Association; past member and chair for the Commission on the Accreditation for Marriage and Family Therapy Education; past member and chair for the North Carolina Marriage and Family Therapy Licensure Board

"The WholeFIT program is a toolbox for change. What do you want out of life? I am sure you can pull a tool out of the WholeFIT toolbox to improve or correct what ails you. The WholeFIT program is a no-fluff approach to real change. I have known Jared (W. Jared Dupree) since we were both 'knee-high to a grasshopper,' and I am impressed with his sharing of candid personal life stories in order to help inspire change. I hope you enjoy your pathway to a better life in this book!"

—Brandon J. Hart, MD, licensed pediatrician and neonatologist

"*WholeFIT* is an amazing example of what happens when one brings together leaders in multiple fields with the sole focus of helping individuals achieve a healthier and more balanced approach to living. The practical examples and action items provided throughout the book makes it easy to apply the concepts and ideas discussed. This is the first book that takes a truly wholistic view to one's life, looking at everything from our eating and exercising habits to how we manage finances to how we manage work and relational stressors, and it helps us understand just how interconnected these aspects of our lives really are. A busy professional [myself], spending way too many hours at work, with a wife and four children at home, this book and its wholistic view on life hit the mark for me, as I think it will for many others."

—James C. Billings, PhD, dean, School of Psychology and Marriage & Family Science, Northcentral University

"In a world where we are being bombarded with information, images, and self-proclaimed experts all shouting their expertise of extremes, absolutes, and the latest fads, *WholeFIT: Wellness for Life* provides and promotes clarity, comprehension, and detail from true experts on how to live one's best life. *WholeFIT* is beautifully written for anyone who is looking to find more balance in his or her life with a distinct road map on how to do it. This is a book I will continue to read over and over for myself as well as recommend to all my clients."

—*Miki Eberhardt, BS, registered dietitian nutritionist, NSCA-CPT*

"At some point in our journeys, most of us gain enough life experience to recognize the limitations of 'magic bullet' thinking. We come to understand that one great effort in a single direction will not sustain health or happiness. Instead, we sense the multiple streams of influence flowing around us all the time. I'm grateful to Dr. Jared DuPree and this strong writing team for this volume that stands on the recognition that human beings are integrated creatures. Readers can use this book for making progress toward health in many areas of life, combining for an integrated approach to growth. Thank you, Dr. DuPree and colleagues for such a valuable contribution to the health and wholeness movement."

—*Mark Tidsworth, MDiv, president, Pinnacle Leadership Associates*

"What I like about *WholeFIT* is that it brings everything together in one book. Rather than reading one book on nutrition, another on exercise, and still others on leisure, work, relationships, etc., *WholeFIT* has it all and, most important, shows how a person cannot concentrate on just one area. It takes more work, but to be healthy, one must look at the whole as everything is connected. *WholeFIT* doesn't just give a person a bunch of scholarly information; it also provides action items. It gets the point across that intent to improve is meaningless without action."

—*William H. Meredith, PhD, asociate dean and professor emeritus, Kansas State University*

"*WholeFIT: Wellness for Life* is a comprehensive, well-balanced, and practical handbook! More important, it is more than just a book; it is a word of wisdom written with grace, passion, and integrity. It speaks deep to the heart. Dr. DuPree is a colleague and a dear friend. I have witnessed his life. What he wrote in this book reflects his personhood and lifestyle. This book will give the readers more than just valuable head knowledge, but also courage for a pursuit of transformative life! This book is a real gift—a must-read!"

—*Andrew Imbrie Tezuka, PhD, LCMFT, founder, Life Design Counseling of Japan, faculty, Department of Counseling, Reformed Theological Seminary of Indonesia (STTRI, Indonesia)*

"A few words spring to mind when I think of *WholeFIT*—incredibly insightful, perceptive, expansive and practical. *WholeFIT* is packed full of seamless knowledge of the body with soulful, humanistic wisdom woven in between. It is clear and constructive, while giving achievable solutions to complex problems. The authors offer up a vast amount of knowledge and experience in an organized way that shines a bright light on all parts of health and wellness. This kind of clarity and relevance is certain to be a catalyst for a slew of positive shifts and changes in readers' lives. For readers who are looking to become healthier and happier, *WholeFIT* helps to peel back the layers of overall wellness and connect with a more intuitive, inspired, and expansive self. As a therapist myself, I'm left with an abundance of information and ideas to integrate into the treatment of my own clients. Because *WholeFIT* spans the entire potential of treatment toward overall well-being, its value is enhanced to anyone who is searching for an easy-to-understand, information-packed, and applicable resource."

—*Andrea R. Baker, MA, LMFT, owner of Soul Sesh, WBFF fitness competitor*

"W. Jared DuPree, PhD, offers a wonderful perspective of the systemic nature of wellness. I especially appreciate the attention given to relationships and the relational nature of life. *WholeFIT* values the role of faith and family. In a world that often feels fragmented and disconnected, *WholeFIT* is a voice calling us to live integrated lives that elicit our best in all aspects of who we are and what we do."

—*Kurt Attaway, MA, associate pastor, The Vineyard Church Pearland*

"I loved it. *WholeFIT*'s approach to the focus of balancing every aspect of your life is fresh and right on track. I found the life experiences and examples intriguing, diverse, and inspiring. So few of us recognize how one area of our life is so deeply impacted by other areas of our lives—body does affect leisure, and leisure affects mind, and so on. *WholeFIT* is the perfect guide for defining the needed change and provides the road to get there."

—*Dixie Bullock, coach team manager and certified
professional job search coach, NextJob, Inc.*

"*WholeFIT: Wellness for Life* nailed it! As a licensed social worker, I have witnessed firsthand the importance of assessing and addressing the whole individual to find meaningful and long-term solutions to most of the problems we face as individuals and families. As founder and CEO of See Opportunities and Achieve Results, Inc. Comprehensive Program (SOAR Wellness), I have seen the huge need to assess and address the whole individual when it comes to identifying and solving issues that affect an employee's health and well-being in addition to their performance and productivity on the job. *WholeFIT: Wellness for Life* eloquently illustrates not only the importance of looking at the whole person, but it also gives great practical and easily applied information on how to do it. Anyone looking to make long-term and sustainable positive changes to all aspects of their life should read this book!"

—*Shaun Bills, LSW, CEO, See Opportunities and Achieve Results, Inc. (SOAR)*

"I was so impressed as a therapist reading *WholeFIT: Wellness for Life* because there were many suggestions that offer immediate application for my clients. The way it is written is a perfect blend between the theoretical and the practical. I feel this book is a must-read for those interested in living a more balanced, fulfilled life or as they help others strive to achieve the same."

—*Chad D. Olson, MS, LMFT, clinical director,*
St. George Center for Couples & Families

"*WholeFIT* immediately lit up my mind and fueled my desire to relentlessly pursue a life of wellness in mind, body, and soul. Insights into my own human nature supported by extensive academic and real-world professional experience in physical and mental wellness shines a light onto the path toward wellness by offering an organized, action-oriented approach to this beautiful struggle. This book holds the formula to changing the course of a reactionary, depressed, pleasure-seeking society to one of personal accountability and proactive dedication to wellness. We truly have the power within us to live a life of true joy."

Melinda Yeaman, entrepreneur, XIBA program director for XOJO SPORTS

"'Living well is much more than the absence of disease.'" So states Dr. Jared DuPree, who knows whereof he speaks: While earning his doctorate in human ecology at Kansas State University, DuPree developed theories and approaches that address weight management, chronic illness, and general wellness. But at the age of thirty-one, DuPree—by then a professor at the University of Houston–Clear Lake, and a respected family therapist—learned that he was (literally) a heart attack waiting to happen. Vowing on the spot to transform his life (and share it happily with his wife and small children) DuPree worked his way back to health and fitness through an integrated program emphasizing wellness for body, mind, and soul. Six years later, with the publication of *WholeFIT* DuPree now shares the cumulative expertise of multiple experts in the fields of physical, mental, and spiritual health. Curated with the eye of a behavioral scientist, and accompanied by his own insightful commentary and engaging real-life examples, this comprehensive compendium offers an easy-to-consume guide to creating wellness in ourselves, our relationships with others, and our lives."

—*Marianne L. Hamilton is a Utah-based veteran journalist and content creator,*
and a contributing author for St. George Health & Wellness *magazine, where*
she focuses on the senior demographic. A multiple gold medal–winning athlete
in Senior Games race-walking competitions, she is also a member of the St.
George Arts Commission and active in volunteerism. Along with her husband,
Doug, she is the coadministrator of the St. George Wine Club

"This book has something relevant to everyone. The use of systems theory and interdependence help bring to light how we can find solutions that work for each of us. So often only we know the things that will be easy or hard for us to incorporate in our lives. The approach of this book provides confidence and understanding how to bring that about. With the variety of authors, topics, and examples provided, there is something for everyone in the book. After reading, you'll find at least one example that causes you to think 'Wow I never thought of that' and 'I found something I can try that will work for me.'"

—*John Busch, MBA, entrepreneur*

"W. Jared DuPree shares insights to the enjoyment of an elevated life. Clearly, he expresses that one's joy and happiness is under their control healthily while so many issues and distractions are not: "When we look at what we actually worry about, we find that only a small percentage of our worries are actually in our control." This simple and direct message will help many discover the peace they seek. The concepts that direct you to an improved lifestyle are doable and reachable. *WholeFIT* increases your understanding of manageable life habits that will improve your outlook and results."

—*Jeffrey T. Sherman, Brave Leadership trainer*
and speaker, ShermanSpeaks, LLC

"*WholeFIT: Wellness for Life* is a fantastic book, filled with ideas and helpful information to improve the reader's overall health and wellness. I highly recommend this book because it is insightful and the information shared is simple yet highly effective. Dr. DuPree has written a truly fabulous and life-affirming book, and I believe that it will have a tremendous impact on all who read it."

—*Ever Gonzalez, CEO,* Outlier Magazine *and*
host of the Outlier *On Air podcast*

"I love the approach *WholeFIT* takes in discussing every aspect or area of importance in my life. I have always looked at health as simply exercising and watching what I eat, often neglecting other areas. In reflecting on the ebbs and flows of my own health, I've noticed feeling my better when I am getting along with my wife, but I have never articulated it the way Dr. DuPree does in this book. Great read, great principles to live by."

—*Craig Morris, entrepreneur*

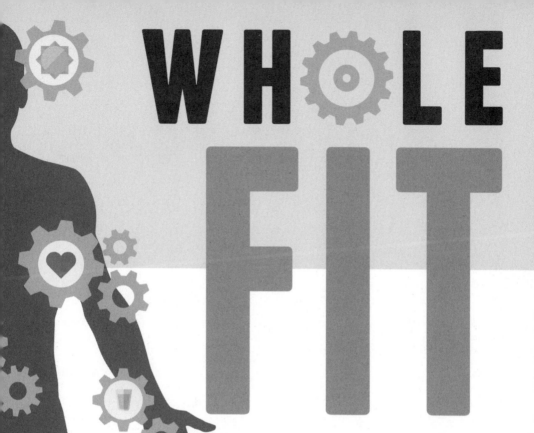

WHOLE
FIT

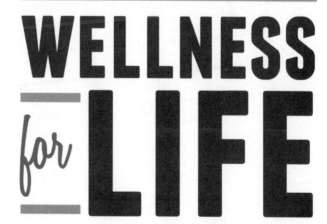

WELLNESS
for LIFE

EDITED BY **W. JARED DUPREE, PhD**

PLAIN SIGHT PUBLISHING
AN IMPRINT OF CEDAR FORT, INC. | SPRINGVILLE, UT

ISBN 13: 978-1-4621-1701-7

Published by Plain Sight Publishing, an imprint of Cedar Fort, Inc.,
2373 W. 700 S., Springville, UT 84663
Distributed by Cedar Fort, Inc., www.cedarfort.com

LIBRARY OF CONGRESS CATALOGING-IN-PUBLICATION DATA
WholeFIT : wellness for life / edited by W. Jared DuPree, PhD.
     pages cm
  Includes bibliographical references.
  ISBN 978-1-4621-1701-7 (perfect bound : alk. paper)
  1. Health. 2. Mind and body. 3. Conduct of life. I. DuPree, W. Jared, 1977- editor.

  RA776.9.W48 2015
  613--dc23

                        2015030133

Cover design by Lauren Error
Cover design © 2015 Cedar Fort, Inc.
Edited and typeset by Eileen Leavitt

Printed in the United States of America

10 9 8 7 6 5 4 3 2 1

Printed on acid-free paper

CONTENTS

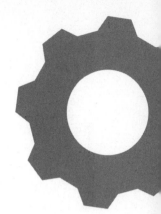

ACKNOWLEDGMENTS

I would like to thank the authors involved in this endeavor. They have dedicated their lives to scholarship and helping others. During each of their journeys, they have discovered treasures of wisdom. We have all been blessed to have unique opportunities that come from serving others professionally, and much of the wisdom comes from helping others as we learn what works and what doesn't.

I would also like to thank Cedar Fort, Inc., for reaching out to me and convincing me to get my ideas on paper. I was giving a speech at Dixie State University, and a representative from the publisher came up to me afterward and told me, "You need to write a book on this." I don't think this book would exist without that nudge.

I would like to acknowledge my mentors throughout the years that have given me the autonomy and encouragement to create through ideas, study and practice. Specifically, the following paved a significant path for my mind or career: Bill Meredith, Candy Russell, Karen Meyers-Bowman, Jeff Hinton, Mark White, Mark Tidsworth, Leslye Mize, and Brent Bradley.

I would like to thank Michael Olson, my partner at the Center for Couples & Families along with the many great managers, therapists, and employees we have had over the years. Mike and his wife have been there with me growing a business based on good principles, which isn't always easy in a down economy. Equally, Mike's passion and creativity in a burgeoning field have greatly added to our development of our WholeFIT approach.

I would like to acknowledge our therapists and behavioral health specialists at the Centers for Couples & Families, along with all helping professionals, including physicians, nurses, dieticians, trainers, psychologists, therapists, social workers, and clergy. You have been in the trenches working with the downtrodden and heartbroken—you have been there with them. Some are physically down, while many are emotionally and spiritually tired. Sometimes, it can be a lonely, burdening place to be in when working with someone that needs you. Thank you for being there for them. You don't get the recognition you deserve.

I would like to thank my own family and friends who have given me great support over the years. I would like to thank my beautiful wife, Anna, and my four wonder children. In many ways, this book is written for me so I can be a better father and husband and take advantage of my greatest asset—my family.

Finally, I would like to thank my many past patients and clients. I have learned so much from you. I feel honored to have participated in your lives even for a short time.

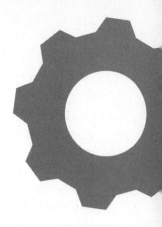

FOREWORD

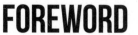

I have spent the majority of my professional career caring for individuals with injuries and pain. Sometimes we have the ability to intervene and take away the pain or medical concern, which is great! Unfortunately, despite our best efforts to help a patient, we fall short, and the patient is left with a constellation of chronic symptoms, which limits the life the patient wants to live and ultimately their quality of life.

On a practical level, I have observed three general factors that impact our risk of developing illness or healing from illness when it occurs:

1. Our environment

2. Professionals

3. Wellness

First, there is the environment where we live which can include public safety, air quality, food sources, disease, events, disasters, or toxic chemicals. We largely don't have much control over these factors at the individual level. However, as communities we can seek to reduce disease through vaccinations, address the quality of air we breathe where we live or work, consider toxic materials exposures through chemicals in our environment, and reduce bacterial exposures through unsuspected food sources. Hopefully, we can continue to improve the health of our environments to help reduce illness.

Second, the innovations and technological advances of modern medicine allow a medical provider to diagnose a disease, medically intervene to rid the body of disease, and engage in medical or surgical interventions when needed. We have come a long way, but there is still much to learn. As providers, we hope for a cure, but more often than not we work to minimize the impact of the disease and its associated symptoms, managing the ailment over time.

Third, we are able to be educated on wellness behaviors and make them a part of our daily lives. It's a simple concept—understand what we can do to make us well and then do it. In reality, our lives get busy and filled with too much stuff, and we neglect our wellness. We don't make the choices that lead to lives filled with wellness behaviors. If we truly understood how our choices and behaviors contributed to wellness or illness, we would pay more attention to this area of our lives. Of all the areas that impact our health, wellness is the area in our lives that we can actually control; we can make changes personally that lead to health.

WholeFIT addresses this third category of health and is a great place to start to understand how to be well through thinking, feeling, and doing. The WholeFIT approach helps the reader understand the connection between thoughts, motivation, and actions. In addition, taking care of our bodies through nutrition and exercise while addressing our relationships, spirituality, and life balance can help readers truly become well in all areas of their lives. The reader who truly engages in this approach will understand that how we choose to live impacts our wellness and will learn practical strategies to incorporate healthy behaviors into our lives.

As a provider, my goal is to help my patients to the best of my abilities. Even though we continue to improve our environment and I continue to hone my skills, I have personally become more and more interested in wellness as I realize all three areas must be addressed to truly be well. I hope you will enjoy these invaluable lessons as much as I have as you read about a topic that could truly save your life in more ways than one.

Jon B. Obray, MD
Board Certified in Pain Medicine
Board Certified in Anesthesiology
Medical Director of Clinical Neurosciences,
Dixie Regional Medical Center,
Intermountain Healthcare Physician,
Southwest Spine and Pain Center

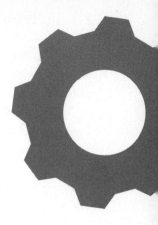

INTRODUCTION

M any years ago, I found myself sitting in an old school building in rural Mississippi amidst humidity, dust, and a group of twelve wide-eyed elementary school kids. Ranging from seven to nine years old, these boys were identified as kids who were struggling. Many were diagnosed with ADHD, some had other mental health disorders, and all had family problems at home. It was a difficult job for me. I was right out of school, determined to help families, but I soon became frustrated as I began to face the realities of the healthcare system, the inequalities of rural America, and the impact of poverty. That frustration soon turned into discouragement and sadness.

As I spoke with these families, I quickly learned that there aren't many "cookie-cutter" answers to today's challenges. Where do I start? Do I coordinate with the physician down the road to help with a mother's diabetes that makes it difficult to keep a job? Do I help the father find a job, knowing that the amount of money coming into the home can't cover the medical bills, let alone food for the children? Do I help the family learn how to de-stress amidst all the problems at school with child A or child B? Do we work on the marriage because it's just hanging on by a thread? Do I blame them for drinking away their problems because I can't see many clear answers myself? So many challenges, so many places to help, so many possible roads.

I realized that all of it is connected. Our health, relationships, finances, nutrition, fitness, emotions, thoughts, past, present and views of the future—it is all connected. That got me thinking.

I left Mississippi because I felt the system was broken and I wanted to go figure it out. I had some tools I learned in graduate school, but organizational constraints didn't really allow me to use them well. Part of the problem was

1

the health-care system, part of it was the economic system, and part of it was our own society and beliefs about change, health, and wellness. I was accepted to a doctoral program that allowed me explore my ideas and think outside of the box. I started working at Mercy Hospital in Manhattan, Kansas, while working on my own research in a place that encouraged discovery. Soon, I began to notice that I wasn't alone in my thinking. There were hints of colleagues and professionals around me who were suggesting that maybe we need to see how fitness impacts emotions or marriage impacts health or nutrition impacts life balance. My first pilot run was to use some of my ideas as we created a weight management program at Mercy Hospital. During the first ten minutes of an initial consultation with a client, we often explored their relationships, finances, businesses, families, and emotions, and found that clients with severe weight management issues did much better if we worked at solving problems in areas not related to weight. Once those issues were tackled, the weight was "magically" easier to manage.

Fast-forward a couple more years. I thought we had great ideas and a great model to help people with their health and wellness. We had evidence suggesting that working on the "whole person" (their health, wellness, nutrition, fitness, life balance, emotions, and so on) was much more successful than treating one area at a time. We also knew from our work and the work of others that not only did this help with weight management, but it was also helpful for dealing with chronic illness, disabilities, and other life challenges. The problem was that our health-care and economic systems were not set up for this type of approach. In fact, most of the time they rejected it. Realizing that I needed to have a clear understanding of the economic drivers that control our health-care system, I packed my wife and children up yet again and moved them cross-country so I could earn an MBA. If I truly wanted to disrupt what I saw as a broken system, I needed to understand how money works, how the economy works, and how the health-care system works.

I left the Darla Moore School of Business with final degree in hand and accepted a position at the University of Houston–Clear Lake. Call it serendipity or coincidence, but a colleague of mine (Dr. Michael Olson) moved in down the road a year later, taking a position at the University of Texas Medical Branch–Galveston as their director of behavioral medicine. We began working on our ideas, applying them in our own practices and with our patients at the University of Texas Medical Branch. We later called the ideas and approach WholeFIT and began working with individuals, providers, and clinics on how to develop a better approach to health and wellness. We both knew at the time that something was happening in health care. Something was happening in how we view change, wellness and patient care. We recognized the rumblings of a nationwide paradigm shift.

This massive shift in mind-set has already begun to have an impact. Shifts in the economy, in our health-care system, and in the attitudes of patients and providers mean that health and wellness is on the verge of taking a different shape. Forces that had their genesis more than two decades ago are now building in velocity. Our wellness professionals (medical and nonmedical) are getting better at working together to consider all aspects of a patient's health (mind, body, soul, and relationships). We are beginning to be able to focus more effectively on how to help people live better and achieve long-term results rather than putting Band-Aids on symptoms that merely cover up the skin-deep splinters without ever digging deeply enough to find the root causes.

Although we are relying on evidence and research, this book is designed to be approachable, relatable, and full of stories and experiences from our own professional lives and lives of others who inspire us. We will address what we feel are the main factors that impact our health and wellness, whether you are hoping to learn how to address weight, chronic illness, being overworked, having difficulty with a troubled teen, experiencing financial distress, or struggling with a different challenge. We'll teach you to analyze not only how all of these areas in your life are interconnected but also how they influence outcomes for one another. The following areas will be addressed:

- Mind: Motivation, Emotions, and Thoughts

- Body: Nutrition, Fitness, and Health

- Relationships: Family, Love, and Spirituality

- Life Balance and Integration: Stress, Community, Work, and Finance

- Health: Wellness and Life Planning

I still think of my experiences in Mississippi and wonder what I could have done differently with what we know now. We aren't quite there yet, but we are much closer. I still think of a little boy and his family from Magee, Mississippi, that could have used what we have to offer today. I think of many of those families and the many that came after. My hope is that we can help today's families open more doors to health and wellness as we address the many important areas of our lives. Our hope is that we can all accept the invitation to be well for life!

Happy trails!

W. Jared DuPree, PhD, MBA

SECTION 1

A COMPREHENSIVE APPROACH TO WELLNESS

*"The whole is greater than
the sum of its parts."*

—*Aristotle* (Metaphysics, *book VIII*)

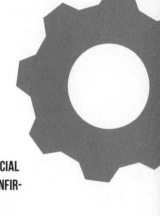

1 **WELLNESS FOR LIFE**

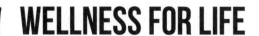

BY W. JARED DUPREE, PHD, MBA

> "HEALTH IS A STATE OF COMPLETE PHYSICAL, MENTAL AND SOCIAL WELL-BEING AND NOT MERELY THE ABSENCE OF DISEASE OR INFIRMITY."[1] —WORLD HEALTH ORGANIZATION

W. JARED DUPREE, PhD, MBA, earned his PhD from Kansas State University, developing theories and approaches that address weight management, chronic illness, and general wellness. He later earned an IMBA (International MBA) from the University of South Carolina, learning how to implement change models in the health-care system and the economy. Jared has worked with many individuals and families on helping them find more happiness and balance in life. He is the founder of the St. George Health & Wellness *magazine (SaintGeorgeWellness.com), the founder of The Center for Couples & Families (Couples-Families.com), the cofounder of WholeFIT (WholeFITwellness.com) and continues to engage in research as an assistant professor at Dixie State University while living with his family in beautiful St. George, Utah. He enjoys mountain biking, traveling, gardening, and spending time with his family.*

Six years ago, I was told if I didn't make some changes, I would die young. I was thirty-one years old, married with three children, working as a professor at the University of Houston–Clear Lake, and seeing clients as a family therapist at night. I played basketball once or twice a week and lifted weights off and on. I drank soda occasionally, ate like the average American (so-so), and served in my local church. Life was good, I thought. One Saturday afternoon in November (I tended to get sick a lot in November) I headed to the urgent care because I was coughing so much it was hard to sleep, and I felt like it might be bronchitis. I thought I would get some antibiotics and be good to go. Unfortunately, after the doctor checked my breathing, oxygen levels, and heart, she immediately announced she wanted to admit me to the hospital. Because I didn't want to pay the high ER fees that come with a visit—often $1,400 or more—I had to convince her that I would make an appointment with a cardiologist the following Monday. She seemed worried to let me go.

After several visits to the cardiologist, a stress test, and some ultrasounds, a grim-faced doctor said to me, "You see all those people sitting in the waiting room? They are thirty years older than you—some more than that. There is no reason you should be here at your age, but here you are. You need to make some changes or you won't be around very long." I was stunned. I guess I fit the stereotype of physicians and providers of old—we don't always take care of ourselves like we do our own patients and clients! This wake-up call was what I needed to make some changes that improved not only my health but also my life!

Today, I am learning personally that everything is connected. My concern about our finances impacts my stress, which impacts the way I eat, which impacts my energy levels and my desires to exercise, which make me more injury-prone, which influences what hobbies I engage in or don't, which leads to feelings of depression at times, which impacts my relationship with my wife and kids and my own spirituality, and so on. I'm guessing some of you have similar stories. At the same time, I realize that as I balance my life (eliminating overwork) and make time for exercise, I tend to eat better, feel better, and have better energy levels. This impacts my mood and my relationship with my wife and kids, which leads to greater feelings of self-worth and more connection to my spirituality. Both examples are shortened versions of an even more complex, systemic picture of how each of the elements of my life is connected.

Even though I was motivated in the past to help my patients and clients with their own health, life balance, and life enjoyment, today I'm even more motivated to help my own life, especially as I consider my greatest asset: my family. You look at life very differently when your eighteen-month-old daughter looks up at you with a big smile, dimples, and a sparkle in her eye or a four-year-old boy reaches for your hand, excited about life as you head outside. I want to live a well life for me and also for my family.

The subtitle of this book has a double meaning. "Wellness for life" suggests a desire to be well, but it also suggests being well for your whole life. In other words, this book is not about quick fixes or fad diets or suggestions that are unrealistic or flat out don't work. We want to share with you principles and patterns of living a well life, which includes how we treat our bodies, minds, emotions, and relationships. This includes living well within the context of our home, workplace, places of worship, community, society, and world. "Wellness for life" also has another meaning for me, and some of you may find a similar motivation. I'm doing this for my life, literally. I don't want to die young, let alone live a life that does not provide me and my family with the ability to enjoy one another and what this world offers. In addition, even if my life was not at stake, I don't know if living with low energy, low motivation, and in avoidable pain amidst distant relationships is the best use of my time and place on this earth. In other words, "wellness for life" is an invitation to us all to be well so that we can enjoy life to the fullest and live a life that helps us connect with others, maximize our talents and strengths, and be good to the bodies that have been given to us.

Our goal has been to create a book that will cause a domino effect of positive change in the lives of every reader. For this reason, we've written this book to be

1. Approachable: we want to share stories, experiences, case studies, and examples to help illustrate principles.

2. Practical: we want to share information that can be used and applied.

3. Informative: we want to share information that is research-based when possible, using language that is easily understood.

I hope this book can be helpful for you. I hope what we offer and suggest is realistic. I hope what we share can make a difference in your own life and in your relationships. Let the wellness begin!

WHAT IS IMPORTANT IN OUR LIVES?

Let me take you back to the experience I shared at the beginning of the chapter. Consider yourself in my shoes: what would you think about if you were told you may not live very long? Most of us faced with a grim diagnosis think first of our families. Who would teach my son to shoot a basketball if I wasn't around? I thought about my girls; who would show them an example of being a good man? I thought about my wife. She is a kind, tender person who doesn't let too many people get close to her. Would my death take the sparkle out of her eye? Would she ever get it back? Would someone be there to comfort her? Would she allow herself to be comforted by others? Our relationships are one of our most important assets in this life, and when faced with a diagnosis that tells us life is ending, most of us immediately think more about relationships and less about possessions.

What does it mean to be healthy? What does it mean to be well? Are we healthy enough to engage in daily activities of survival and comfort (walking, taking a shower, fixing a meal, sleeping restfully, and so on)? Are we healthy enough to engage beyond activities of survival and enjoy our lives? In other words, do we have the motivation and energy to engage in hobbies, exercise, play with our kids or grandkids, learn, connect with others, and serve?

Health is often associated with our physical bodies while wellness is often associated with an approach to living. However, even these two concepts have started to intertwine. Consider the following definition by the World Health Organization: "Health is a state of complete physical, mental, and social well-being and not merely the absence of disease or infirmity."

When our health and wellness are going "well," we are able to engage in our daily activities and pursue long-term goals. A healthy body, mind, and set of relationships allow us to more fully enjoy life. We can get up, feel rested, eat, shower, work, play, and connect. Beyond the basics of life, we can learn, grow, pursue our passions, engage in hobbies, be active, be restful, love, forgive, and progress. At the other end of the spectrum, if we face disease, ailments, or problems in living, it can become difficult to enjoy life or to be independent. Obviously, there are conditions that are out of our control due to genetics, accidents, unavoidable diseases, and, yes, old age. The key principle to consider is that our health and wellness are important aspects of our lives because they give us the chance to more fully live our lives.

Finally, many of my patients and clients will drift toward an exploration of personal passions, motivations, identity, and even life purpose. They ask themselves, "What am I meant to do in this life?" or "What brings me the most joy?" I remember working with a woman in her seventies asking the same questions: "I have lived for so long doing this or that, yet I still believe I haven't found my true place. I believe there is much to discover and much to offer. I'm excited to discover that for me." No matter the age, income, race, ethnicity, or religion, many want to know their place in the world, how they fit, and what they have to offer.

As we consider what is important in our lives, we begin to understand that if we get caught up in trying to achieve empty goals, we'll likely end up feeling empty. The wise man or woman who realizes what is important in life and lives to achieve the important will likely end up feeling peace—peace with themselves, with others, and with God or a higher power.

The areas considered most important in life can usually be distilled down to these three:

1. Our relationships: our relationship with ourselves, with others and with a higher power

2. Our health: our physical, mental, emotional, spiritual, and social well-being

3. Our life purpose: our motivations, talents, strengths, and beliefs and sharing them with the world

WHAT FACTORS INFLUENCE WELLNESS?

As my partner and I developed the WholeFIT approach, our focus was to help patients address all the factors that impact wellness. We relied on research and our clinical experience in developing some visual models of what to consider when assessing and assisting patients. As seen in Figure 1, we believe the following areas are important factors to review when considering what may be impacting a person's wellness: our bodies (health, fitness, and nutrition), our minds (motivations, mindfulness, and learning), our emotions (self-esteem, coping skills, and healing), our relationships (self, others, and higher power), leisure (play, fun, and hobbies), career (fit, performance, work balance, and finances), and our community (social, spiritual, professional, and resources). We believe that to fully live well, we each need to consider how these areas impact our lives. As we will discuss further, all of these areas are deeply connected to one another. Change in one impacts change in other areas.

Figure 1: Wellness Areas

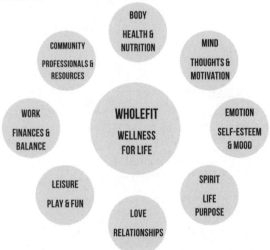

The second set of diagrams is used to provide the framework behind our approach. (See Figure 2.) We will discuss some of these areas in upcoming chapters. After chapter 2, we will discuss how our individual thoughts, emotions, motivations, and sense of life purpose impact our health and wellness in chapters 3, 4, 5, and 6. These individual patterns influence how we see the world and what drives us. Equally, our thoughts and emotions impact our health patterns as they relate to fitness, nutrition, illness, and general health, which will be discussed in chapters 7 through 11. Our individual and health patterns are influenced by our relationships, including our connection with a spouse or partner, our families, and our connection to a higher power (spirituality). We will discuss how our relationships impact our overall wellness in chapters 12 through 14. Finally, our individual patterns, health behaviors, and relationships are connected to how we integrate and balance our different roles as they relate to a career, finances, education, and overall stress management. We will discuss ways to address life balance and the different roles we have in chapters 15 through 17. Finally, we will put everything together and give some examples of how to address different challenges using a comprehensive, systemic wellness approach in chapter 18.

Figure 2: Framework for WholeFIT approach

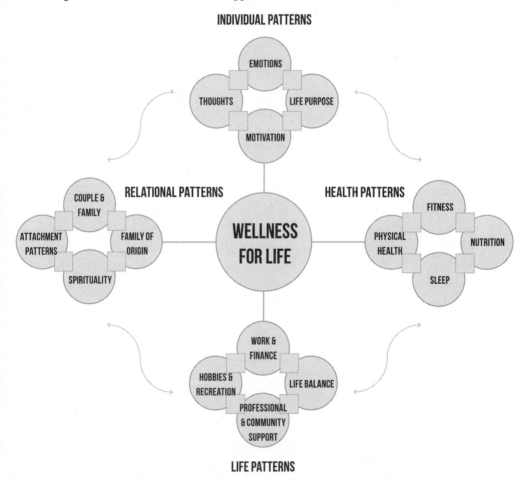

We want you to be aware that living well is much more than the absence of disease. Living well is considering the important people and parts of our lives and making the most of what is given to us. Living well is learning to live in a manner that takes advantage of our talents and strengths. We learn to find the path that not only makes the most sense but also brings the most peace because we are true to ourselves and others. Our bodies, minds, and souls will respond as we find more peace and direction in our lives.

⚙ ACTION ITEMS

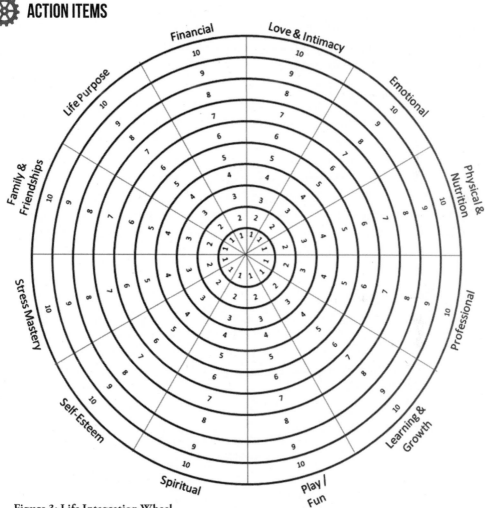

Figure 3: Life Integration Wheel

INSTRUCTIONS

1: COMPLETE THE INTEGRATION WHEEL WITH THE LAST THREE MONTHS IN MIND; ESPECIALLY FOCUS ON THE LAST THREE WEEKS.

2: REMEMBER, THE GOAL IS NOT TO HAVE ALL "10'S," RATHER, CONSIDER THE AREAS THAT ARE BOTH ABOVE AND BELOW "6." THESE ARE YOUR STRONG AREAS AND AREAS OF NEED.

3: CONSIDER HOW EACH AREA IMPACTS THE OTHERS.

ASSESSMENT KEY

0 = COMPLETELY LACKING IN MY LIFE

1 = NEARLY NOTHING

2 = VERY MUCH LACKING IN MY LIFE

3 = ONLY A LITTLE BIT

4 = COULD BE BETTER, BUT GETTING BY

5 = NEUTRAL, NEITHER GOOD NOR BAD

6 = ADEQUATE LEVEL IN MY LIFE

7 = I'M CONTENT WITH WHAT I HAVE

8 = I'M MORE THAN CONTENT

9 = GENEROUS ABUNDANCE IN MY LIFE

10 = IT CAN'T GET ANY BETTER THAN THIS

Begin by filling out a Life Integration Wheel (© 2015, all rights reserved. Originally developed by Glenn Norman, MA and W. Jared DuPree, PhD, MBA). We used to call it the Life Balance Wheel but discovered that people assumed that you needed to be equally balanced among all areas, and this is not necessarily the case. You will put more energy in some areas and less energy in others based on your current needs.

As you fill out the wheel, consider the last three months of your life or less. See the assessment key and instructions box listed with Figure 3 for more details. The goal is not to be at a perfect "10" in each area, rather we would hope most areas were at a "6" with the understanding that some may be a little lower or higher. A "6," as the key suggests, represents an "adequate level in my life" of whatever area you are considering. If you are below a "6," we hope that the chapters in this book will give you some ideas that could help enhance those areas. You may also consider seeking out the guidance of a professional if needed. Chapter 18 discusses ways to use the wheel and the other principles mentioned in this book to develop a plan for your wellness. Knowing where you are at in the different areas of your life is a good place to start. For now, fill out the wheel so you know which areas you need to maintain, which areas may need additional support or change, and which areas are strengths.

CONCLUSION

The upcoming chapters are designed to help give you some perspective of the myriad factors that impact our health and wellness. While it's impossible to cover everything, we hope to give you some important "nuggets" of information that we think will be most helpful. We will also give you action items in each chapter to consider so you can begin to apply some of these areas. So, if you are ready to take steps to become the healthiest and happiest you've been in a long time (maybe the healthiest and happiest you've ever been), let's get started!

NOTE

1. "Preamble to the Constitution of the World Health Organization as adopted by the International Health Conference," New York, 19–22 June, 1946, Official Records of the World Health Organization, no. 2 (entered into force on April 7, 1948), 100.

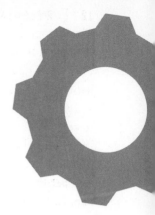

2 EVERYTHING IS CONNECTED

BY BRANDEN HENLINE, PHD

"LEARN HOW TO SEE. REALIZE THAT EVERYTHING CONNECTS TO EVERYTHING ELSE."[1] —LEONARDO DA VINCI

BRANDEN HENLINE *holds a PhD in marriage and family therapy from Texas Tech University and is a Clinical Fellow and Approved Supervisor with the American Association for Marriage and Family Therapy (AAMFT). He is a professional member and Certified Family Life Educator (CFLE) with the National Council on Family Relations (NCFR). Dr. Henline is a Licensed Marriage and Family Therapist (LMFT) in Arizona and Utah and has maintained an active clinical practice since fall 2000. As a therapist, he has worked with families and children, adolescents, couples, and individuals on issues related to parenting, behavioral problems, self-harm, depression, anxiety, eating disorders, trauma, conflict resolution, infidelity, pornography, addiction recovery, intimacy development, and strengthening marriage and family relationships. Dr. Henline has built his career on training other therapists. He is the founding program director for the family therapy training programs at Northcentral University (NCU) and now works as the director of clinical field placements. Many of the nearly 1300 students who attend the program come from rural areas where there is a dearth of qualified family services providers. His work will impact millions of people through the clients these therapists will serve over the years. He still maintains an active clinical practice and enjoys supervising and mentoring other therapists. Dr. Henline is married and he and his wife have four children together. In addition to English, Dr. Henline speaks, reads, and writes Thai.*

INTRODUCTION

Have you ever wondered what causes things to change? Or why it is that change is so hard? Researchers, therapists, and theorists have established a lot of ideas about how change occurs. As a young college student, I thought I had it figured out. (Oh, the hubris of being young!) Change, I thought, was simple. The short version of my philosophy of change was that a person simply needed to decide what they wanted in a given situation, choose to act the way that was needed for the desired outcome and, voilà!, it would happen. Said another way, in situation A, choice B will lead to outcome C, or A + B = C. Even in my classes, I was taught about behaviorism and the idea that stimulus + response = outcome. It seems logical enough, right?

At the time, my parents were struggling in their marriage, and I was confident that I could use my approach to help them resolve their differences. I sat the two of them down, clarified that what they should want is to be happily married, and explained that what they needed to do was be nice, communicate better, and go out on dates more consistently. I sent them away with this magically simple solution with the hope that they would follow my advice and all would be well. Not surprisingly, they never talked to me about their marital problems again. Rather, they finalized their divorce less than a year later.

On a more positive note, I kept studying, and I learned that life and change are not nearly as simple as I had once believed. As I finished college, I made the decision to pursue graduate training to become a marriage and family therapist and have learned much more effective methods to help people improve their relationships. I can trace the decision to become a family therapist to a turning point I experienced in a family science class I completed as a general education requirement. The professor of the class taught about a philosophy known as systems theory. Rather than seeing life's outcomes as a simple matter of cause and effect or choice and consequences (think A + B = C), he taught that everything is part of a system that changes or stays the same based on mutual influence among all of the parts. Said another way, A, B, C, D, and E are all tied together and, because of their connection to each other, they will experience a given outcome F or G, depending on the way they interact. Further, systems have certain tendencies, and understanding these tendencies can help us to maintain things the way they are and find ways to create change in a system.

One example that helped me to understand the idea of systems is to consider the parts of a watch or clock. Which part of a clock causes it to work? Is it the spring? Maybe it is the second hand, the minute hand, or the hour hand? Or, maybe it is the series of moving cogs inside the clock that we do not really see? Clearly, all of the parts of a clock work together to cause the whole clock to function the way that it does. The same is true with the motor on your car. If the alternator or the fan belt cease to function, the entire engine will eventually shut down. The same is true in families, in our health, and in the systemic nature of our lives. Truly, everything is connected!

Think of this in your own life. If you are seeking to improve your health, consider how your relationships affect what happens in your physical health. Some interactions are soothing, encouraging, exciting, rewarding, and motivational and lead us to think, feel, and act in healthy ways. Does an argument cause weight gain or ulcers or reckless behavior? Probably not directly, and not just one argument. But we do know that a pattern of conflict results in higher stress hormones in the body which, over time, can result in poor functioning in our digestive system, our immune system, and even our logical thoughts and decision making. In this way, what is happening in our family system can have a significant impact on what is happening with the internal systems of our body and result in unwanted health outcomes. Yet, the same is true of positive relationship experiences, which can promote lower stress and result in more health-promoting behaviors.

The connection between relationships and health is only one example of the mutual impact that systems can have in our lives. All of our systems are connected. The focus of this chapter is on learning to see these connections and use them to your advantage to facilitate greater health and wellness. Understanding these connections will allow you to see life from a new perspective. Rather than A + B = C thinking, you will begin to see the interconnections in all things. This rich and broad "systems" perspective has benefited my own life, my relationships, my health, and my professional work. I am confident that it can make a difference in your approach to your own health and wellness.

SYSTEMS THEORY CONCEPTS

Levels of Systems

Our life experiences are inherently a result of connections between multiple levels of systems. We live as individuals within a family system or a system of friends or even coworkers. This small system is part of a larger community or a work organization. Our communities are part of societies within larger cities, regions, states, or nations. Beyond that, we are all part of a world community or system. We can even see the systems that make up the atmosphere, habitats, and ecosystems within our planet Earth. Our Earth is part of our larger solar system, which is part of our galaxy, which is part of the larger system we refer to as the known universe.

Just as we as individuals are part of larger and larger systems within the universe, we can also see progressively smaller microsystems within ourselves. Our bodies are made up of digestive systems, nervous systems, circulatory systems, reproductive systems, immune systems, skeletal systems, and so on. These systems are made up of smaller parts that function as a system. The heart, as an example, is made up of multiple muscles, ventricles, valves, vessels, and tissues that function together to pump our blood. These organs and body parts are made up of cells that function as systems. Even cells are made up of atoms that also are mini systems of electrons, protons and neutrons.

The importance of thinking about these layers and levels of systems is that doing things to impact one system can result in changes in other parts of the system. Changing salt intake, for example, can affect cell functioning, the circulatory system, and water retention in the body. Similarly, doing service in your community can inspire others, create new opportunities for service, increase your sense of making a contribution, improve your spirituality, and reduce stress.

Knowing and seeing the levels of systems can help us be aware of the influences in our lives and opportunities we have to make changes for the better. Consider bike-friendly towns like Portland, Oregon. Because many people in that community value riding bikes, they are all are active in riding to work or riding recreationally. With time and persistence, these riders have had success getting the local government to add more bike lanes, create mass transit that supports bike riders, and enact laws and community efforts to maintain and increase efforts to keep Portland bike-friendly. Both cycling enthusiasts and people who do not ride at all are all affected by the systemic changes that have occurred in Portland.

Change in one system or sub-system can create change in other parts of the system. For example, if I respond to criticism or conflict with kindness, forgiveness or service, I may experience less stress, better sleep, better digestion, and overall better health. What happens in the larger system impacts the smaller systems and vice versa.

Interdependence

Once you start to see and understand different types and levels of systems, a major concept to keep in mind is the notion of interdependence. Change in part of a system changes the system. To illustrate, imagine standing in a circle with a group of four or five friends, with each person having his or her hands tied to the person on either side. In such a scenario, if one person fell to the ground, the others in the group would be pulled in the same direction, perhaps resulting in the whole group collapsing to the floor. Similarly, if one or more people in the group started moving in a given direction, everyone else would have to move that direction with them or else exert influence to keep the movers back with the group in the original location. What happens to one person in this connected group affects the others in the group just like moving one object in a mobile over a baby's crib will move all of the other objects.

In systems theory, understanding interdependence helps us to see that the experiences of one person or one part of a system are not isolated ineffectual occurrences. A father's drinking behaviors can adversely impact all members of a family. A sibling's success or misbehavior at school can have ripple effects on others in the family for years to come. If we are thinking only on the individual level, systems theory still applies. Proactive healthy nutritional choices can result in higher, consistent energy levels, improved fitness and enhanced brain functioning. Parts of systems do not function in isolation.

There are many examples of this wholeness or interdependence in health behaviors. Consistency with exercise improves sleep. Eating junk food can make you lethargic and uninterested in exercise. In medical settings, improved relationships result in greater treatment compliance, positive treatment outcomes, lower medical costs, and long-term resilience. Proper hydration improves weight loss efforts, emotional regulation, brain functioning, exercise, and nutrition. Research shows that people with workout partners are more consistent and successful in health improvement efforts. Why? The importance of the relationship improves accountability, motivation, and rewards associated with being healthy.

Because of interdependence, there are many potential assets to support health and wellness. Recognizing and addressing multiple aspects of your health systems (relationships, nutrition, exercise, spirituality, community involvement, and friendships) can create compounding benefits to spark and maximize wellness outcomes. Remember, change in one part of the system changes the system. As such, there is no need to worry about changing everything at once. Instead, just start somewhere and let your efforts build momentum across your systems, like a stone thrown into a pond that causes far-reaching ripple effects.

Entropy

Entropy is a systems-theory term that refers to the tendency that all systems, if left alone, will fall into greater disorder over time. Scientists believe that the universe is spinning into greater disarray. An object left out in the dirt will eventually break down or decompose and no longer be recognizable as what it once was. If we do not work to strengthen our friendships or family relationships, we become distant and disconnected with each other. If we do not work our muscles, they will atrophy and wither away.

As part of my professional life, I work as a family therapist. To drive this concept of entropy home, I like to offer an analogy to my clients about a bicycle on a hill. If you are riding a bike up a hill, whether steep, moderate, or minor in slope, as long as you keep pedaling, you will stay upright and moving in a forward direction. But if you do not pedal, you will slow down, lose momentum, potentially fall over and get injured, or face the need to turn around and let gravity pull you downhill. By nature, entropy, like gravity, has the effect of pulling things apart.

However, in the face of entropy, a little work can be useful in keeping up the momentum to maintain success in our lives. It is easier to stay healthy than to recover from poor health. It is easier to keep engaging in healthy behaviors and relationships once we get things started. As quoted by Ralph Waldo Emerson, "That which we persist in doing becomes easier for us to do; not that the nature of the thing itself is changed, but that our power to do is increased."

I saw this capacity to overcome entropy in my life as I learned to be a distance runner. In 2006, I saw the need to improve my health, and the least-expensive option was to start running. When I first started, my effort to become a runner involved intermittent walking (and wheezing) in between efforts to jog as far as possible before needing to walk again. As I recall, the first time I "ran" 3 miles, it took me just over 38 minutes. That is just under 13 minutes per mile or about 4.5 miles per hour. In contrast, professional marathon runners maintain a pace of 5- to 6-minute miles (roughly 10–12 miles per hour) for 26.2 miles.

When I first started running up to 3 miles at a time, I didn't anticipate running greater distances. However, a year or so later, I had a conversation with a good friend who had finished a marathon, and that planted a seed in me. The discussion with my friend motivated me to want to run more and finish a marathon for myself. Over the next couple of years, I completed a 10k (6.2 miles), a half marathon (13.1 miles), and then two full marathons. As I kept running, I made improvement against the entropy that would have resulted from inactivity. Rather than falling apart over time or experiencing worse and worse health, I put effort into being a little better. It became easier to do, and I found that I really enjoy running. It has resulted in motivation, improved health, and connections with family and friends who I have run and trained with. By nature, life and time will build you up or break you down, depending on whether you choose to invest in your health or give in to the inevitable impact of entropy.

Paul Watzlawick, one of the early pioneers of family therapy, is quoted as saying "One cannot not communicate." Similarly, a person cannot not feel. And, we cannot not behave. Every day, we each make decisions about what we will say, feel, and do. Our words, feelings, and actions inevitably lead to the experiences and outcomes of our day. We are always communicating by what we say or do not say. Even giving someone the "silent treatment" is a process of communicating something to another person. Relating to entropy (the tendency of things toward disorder), it is important to consider what we communicate, feel, and do in our daily lives. Left to chance, our words, feelings, and actions will tend to result in distance, damage, and dissatisfaction. But this does not have to be the case. If we realize the impact of entropy in our lives, health, and relationships because we are going to communicate, feel, and act one way or another each day, we can choose to act in meaningful and productive ways.

One poignant lesson I learned in life relating to the impact of entropy occurred in summer 2014 as I sat on a stage as a senior leader among the faculty at a graduation ceremony for Northcentral University. The commencement speaker was Rich Karlgaard, a best-selling author, journalist, and publisher for *Forbes Magazine*. The premise of his speech was a review of lessons he had learned from years of exposure to übersuccessful people. One point that he made really stuck with me. He talked about people like Warren Buffet and Bill Gates and stated that these successful people make a point to get what you have always gotten, always invest, and never spend or consume.

Mr. Karlgaard gave several examples and explained that we can invest our time, money, resources, and energy in things that will have lasting value. Or we can spend our time and resources on fleeting things that are consumed as a result. This idea of investing and not consuming left me thinking about my time with my family, the use of my energy across a day, and even the food I eat. Do I spend my time in silence watching TV or scrolling through social media, or do I invest my time in meaningful connection and memory building with my wife and kids? Do I let distractions and less important tasks consume my energy across a day, or do I invest the effort needed to accomplish prioritized goals each day? Do I consume foods that give temporary satisfaction in return for long-term health complications, or do I invest what is needed to find, prepare, and eat nutrient-rich meals that are satisfying and congruent with my health goals? In short, do I take the path of least resistance and let entropy gradually take its toll in my life and leave me worse off, or do I live purposefully and proactively to pursue improvements and invest in the life I want each day? For me, the decision is clear: it is always best to invest and not spend or consume. In life, we are always either getting better or worse. We will expend our time and energy one way or another. Choose to invest, not spend.

Homeostasis

Homeostasis is a tendency of systems to want to stay the same or maintain the status quo. Perhaps the clearest example of homeostasis is seen in the function of a thermostat in a home. If you set the thermostat at a specific temperature, when things change in the home, such as increased sunlight or higher temperatures outside, the air conditioning turns on to return the home to the desired temperature, perhaps seventy-two degrees. Similarly, if it is cold outside and the doors are left open, when the system notices that the interior temperature has dropped, the heater is turned on to bring the home back up to seventy-two degrees.

We see homeostasis in the internal systems of our bodies. Our heart tends to beat at a steady resting heart rate, which can vary from person to person but often remains the same for an individual over time. When things happen that change our heart rate, such as getting scared or exercising, our bodies begin to do things to return our heart to its resting heart rate. We breathe heavier, slow down, calm down, or get out of situations that allow us to slow our heart and return to our comfortable level of functioning.

Homeostasis occurs in bigger systems such as families and communities as well. Families tend to have patterns of interaction that are their standard or comfortable ways of interacting. Some families are distant; others experience regular conflict and arguments; some spend a lot of time together; and some families have regular routines and traditions that they engage in. These are all examples of homeostasis. The system tends to stay the same over time.

Homeostasis is important to consider in your efforts to improve your health and wellness. When we try to change, there is a tendency to change back to what we are used to. This is seen in the lives of people that make significant changes in their weight but then return to old habits and change back to their old status of being overweight. Some people seek to change but experience pressure from family and friends to return to old patterns. But if you know about homeostasis, you can realize that there is a tendency to return to old default behaviors and you can choose to create new defaults. Realizing that this pressure or tendency is there can help you be aware and choose to be different and stay different. If you always do what you have always done, you will always get what you have always gotten. Said another way, if you start doing what you used to do, you will start getting the same results you used to get.

Aside from recognizing the pressure to return to old patterns, you can use the concept of homeostasis to purposefully create a "new normal" in your life and your family system. Returning to the thermostat analogy, if you are used to keeping your home at seventy-two degrees but decide that seventy-five will be better, you can set the thermostat to seventy-five and work with your

Easy to slip into old habits [handwritten margin note]

family to keep it there. There may be a tendency to reset things to seventy-two. You would have to get used to living at seventy-five and make a purposeful and active decision to maintain the settings at seventy-five degrees. Over time, it will be easier to leave it there.

If someone in your family has been diagnosed with diabetes, it will result in a need to change routines, eating habits, and other health-related behaviors. Because of homeostasis in systems, there will be a tendency to start out with good intentions and eat really healthy meals for a week, and then regress back to doing things the way you always have. But doing so would maintain problems that keep a person with diabetes from getting better or maintaining their health as well as possible. As examples, continuing to drink soda with meals or living sedentary lives would exacerbate the difficulties of regulating blood sugar levels and maintaining the circulation that is needed to stay healthy. Homeostasis is the pressure to not change. But seeing the tendency to maintain homeostasis can help a person or family to be deliberate and change to create a new normal that the family can support.

Positive versus Negative Feedback

All of our words, behaviors and experiences work together to either change our lives or keep them the same. In systems theory, these words and behaviors are referred to as feedback. Everything we do and all that happens to keep our health, relationships, and lives the same is known as *negative feedback* or *change-reducing feedback*. On the other hand, *positive feedback* includes all of the efforts that occur to create change. The words *positive* and *negative*, in this regard, are not about whether you like the feedback or not or whether it is kind, mean, productive, or critical. Rather, positive means that it promotes change and negative feedback diminishes or reduces the likelihood of change.

Understanding positive and negative feedback in systems is useful in your efforts to create or prevent change. You can start to see experiences, words, and interactions with others in terms of whether they are supporting or discouraging change you want in your life. When you see the difference, you can choose to focus on those things that support your efforts.

As a couple and family therapist, the way I have used the concept of positive and negative feedback with clients is to teach them what I call the "talk rule." The talk rule is this: That which is talked about most tends to happen the most. Many clients that start therapy spend much of the time in initial sessions talking about the struggles they are facing and all of the things they recognize that are contributing to the problems. The challenge with this is that this effort maintains the focus on what is not wanted. This is often needed

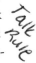

in therapy, to address the concerns that bring people to the office in the first place, build trust and empathy, and set the stage for what needs to be done to work toward improvements. But if you spend all of your time talking about what you do not want, you stay stuck with what you do not want.

In contrast, if you put your time, words, energy, and actions into exploring and acting on goals and behaviors that you do want, these desired outcomes will be your focus, and you will start seeing and doing those things more in your life. Do you want to focus on or increase your problems or undesirable outcomes in life, or do you want new opportunities and healthy results? What do you talk about most: what you *do* want or what you *do not* want? I have found that when we focus on what we do want, we tend to make more progress in life.

Focus on what you do want!

Consider the following examples: A couple may be frustrated about their relationship and have a pattern of complaining or arguing about things that bother them. "You work so much that you are too worn out to do anything with me." "Whenever I come home, you get on my case about everything I didn't do!" In contrast, consider the following alternative comments. "You can be so creative with your work. I'm looking forward to a little creativity with you this evening!" "It is nice to be able to be with you and just relax together sometimes."

To use positive and negative feedback in your own life, choose what you want to change in your life and also those things that you want to maintain the way they are. Then, do things that focus on making the changes you want to make. Look for, embrace, and use words, ideas, and behaviors that create the desired changes. In other words, pay attention to and use positive or change-enhancing feedback to your advantage. If you want to have more energy throughout your day, look for, talk about, and eat foods with genuine nutritional value. If you desire improved spiritual connections in your life, put some time into meditation, read and ponder scriptures, participate in worship services, or learn more about and participate in meaningful personal prayer.

On the other hand, if you have made desired changes in your life and now want to maintain new habits or patterns, spend your time, words, and actions on keeping things the way you now want them. In systems terms, use negative feedback to reduce change from the new normal or homeostasis you have established in your life. Tell your story to others to share about changes you have made to improve your life. Think about and savor the details of what your life is like with the changes. As an example, when I first started running, it was tiring and there were days that I just didn't feel like going. But I started paying attention to how I felt when I finished a run. It was a relief to be done, for sure. But, I also realized that I felt energized, healthy, and powerful when I finished a good running session. The same is true with other forms of exercise and other healthy behaviors. Imagine the difference in how you feel when you have eaten a well-portioned, healthy meal as opposed to how you feel when you overload on too much sugar. Once you have made changes and created a new pattern in your life, paying attention to how you feel and the success you have can help you sustain the change.

1st Order Change versus 2nd Order Change

The last concept from systems theory that I want to emphasize is the difference between short-term and long-term change. The technical terms for these different types of change are 1st order and 2nd order change. As you might expect, short-term, or 1st order change, tends to happen before long-term, or 2nd order, change. When things need to change or improve in life, we typically start with small, surface level changes. Our doctor may give us a directive to reduce our salt, sugar, or fat intake or to get more exercise. If we follow the doctor's advice, we may start with putting away the saltshaker or eat at home instead of stopping for fast food. These changes may result in initial changes in our blood pressure, cholesterol, or weight. But they will not persist or result in greater changes unless we make additional changes. Yet we have to start somewhere. That is why these concepts of 1st and 2nd order change are important. We can start small (with a 1st order change) and then keep the ball rolling by adding to it with a 2nd order change.

In a world that often focuses on bigger and better, quick fixes, multitasking, and immediate gratification, efforts to change can be sabotaged by trying to do too much too soon. Sometimes, a monumental goal or task is too overwhelming, to the point that people choose to do nothing rather than seek to improve. We yield to homeostasis and entropy rather than putting effort into purposeful change. For this reason, I like to encourage people to work on taking "one small step for man" (a 1st order change) rather than a "giant leap for mankind" (more difficult 2nd order change)

Experience shows that people who set one or two goals typically achieve all of them. If we set three or four goals to work on at the same time, we often achieve one or two of them. But if we set five or more goals to focus on simultaneously, often none of them are accomplished. These lessons from the goal-setting literature highlight the value of 1st order and 2nd order changes. When we identify the need to change, if we choose one or two things to work on to get started, we are not so overwhelmed. We have the mental and physical capacity to focus and start to see meaningful results. Knowing what we know about systems and homeostasis, if we stop there, life and circumstances will often turn this initial change and progress around and return us to the way things used to be. But understanding the need for 2nd order change can help you to set new goals and pursue additional changes that result in lasting success.

Yo-yo dieting is a great example of 1st order efforts that never result in lasting change. In contrast, 2nd order change occurs when you make sustainable, realistic changes to the way you live your life. Dieting rarely lasts (1st order change). Making healthy changes to our nutrition, fitness, and life balance that we can truly embrace will lead to long-term change (2nd order change). 2nd order changes lead to more health and wellness rather than trying to lose a certain amount of pounds. The purpose of 2nd order change is to change the "way" we live which will lead to benefits in many areas including our weight

Similarly, whether you have goals for weight loss, improved health, greater simplicity, professional success, or other meaningful changes, you can use these systems principles of 1st and 2nd order change to start small and build momentum to gain enough progress for greater changes. If you start with what you can do and don't stop there but continue on and add new healthy habits in your life, 1st order change will lead to long-term 2nd order change. Success begets success.

 ## ACTION ITEMS

In an effort to support beneficial change and health, I wish to recommend several specific action items that can be implemented based on the principles from this chapter. I invite you to use these strategies in your daily lives to pursue the long-term outcomes that you want in life.

1. **Start seeing systems in your life**. Recognize the interconnections between yourself, your partner, your family, your community, and larger systems, as well as the connections between life experiences and the functioning of various systems within your body. How well your systems function will determine your health outcomes.

2. **Create ripples in your life by making doable, positive changes where you can and sustain them to foster change in additional areas of your life.** Do not try to change everything at the same time, but choose one thing and make a consistent change with it. Then, change another thing to create compound improvements. If all you can do is start drinking more water, set a reasonable goal and drink that amount of water each day. When

that is a habit, consider walking or exercising more. If you are a consistent exerciser, consider improving your flexibility, nutrition, or mindfulness and relaxation.

3. **Create a "new normal" by changing the homeostasis in your life and family**. Think about the way you want your system (your life, your family, your health, your way of living with your illness) to be. Then, with a clear vision of what you want, change the settings of your life to support the new vision. Talk to your family and friends about how you want and need things to be. The more you live the new way, the easier it will become. You and others will get used to the new normal, and you will be able to maintain the new healthy pattern.

4. **Use the "Talk Rule" to create the change you want in your life.** Talk about what you do want more than what you do not want. Put your time, energy, words, and focus into the outcomes you want to see happen.

5. **Start with small changes, but do not stop there.** Do not be satisfied with small, superficial changes. They will not last. Once the 1st order, surface-level changes have begun, let them build momentum to create lasting 2nd order changes. To improve your health, start drinking more water, walking, and tracking what you eat. But then, let those experiences develop into learning to cook healthy and satisfying meals, finding fun ways to exercise that you enjoy and will sustain, and forming lifelong healthy habits. To improve your relationship, start by showing interest, expressing more frequent and genuine appreciation, and being responsive to your partner. But then, keep using interest, appreciation, and responsiveness while you learn to really resolve conflict more effectively, build common goals together, and find ways to really connect intellectually, emotionally, spiritually, socially, physically, and sexually. If you need to learn to live better with chronic pain or illness, start by following sound medical advice, taking your meds as prescribed, and giving yourself permission to rest and recover. But then, learn all that you can about proactive ways to address your pain or illness and make long-term changes in your eating habits, lifestyle, and daily routines that will allow you to thrive within the context of your illness. In short, do what you can to start, and then choose to invest the effort to live as well as you can into the future.

CONCLUSION

Everything in life is connected. There are many philosophies in the world found in books and programs that are intended to support greater health and success. Far too often, the ideas that are promoted end up focusing on isolated concepts that may be meaningful but fail to take into consideration the connections between the systems in our lives. Meditation alone is not likely to sustain a person's efforts at pain management. Medication alone will not create lasting change for an individual struggling with severe depression without other systemic changes in the person's life. Rather, adopting a wholistic approach that considers the interdependence of internal and external systems in your life can lead to useful initial changes, followed by longer term changes that can be sustained for lasting improved wellness.

NOTE

1.   Leonardo da Vinci, as quoted on Goodreads.com, accessed October 23, 2015, https://www.goodreads.com/quotes/679908-learn-how-to-see-realize-that-everything-connects-to-everything.

SECTI⚙N 2

OUR MINDS AND OUR HEARTS

*"If you have inner peace, nobody can force
you to be a slave to the outer reality."*

—*Sri Chinmoy* (Peace, *Agni Press, 1995*)

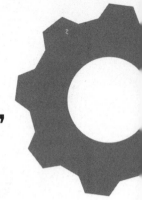

3 AS A MAN AND WOMAN THINKETH AND "FEELETH"

BY W. JARED DUPREE, PHD, MBA

> "THE LAW OF HARVEST IS TO REAP MORE THAN YOU SOW. SOW AN ACT, AND YOU REAP A HABIT. SOW A HABIT AND YOU REAP A CHARACTER. SOW A CHARACTER AND YOU REAP A DESTINY."[1]
> —JAMES ALLEN

As Dr. Henline so beautifully explained in chapter 2, we are all connected both on the inside and out. We are connected to this world through relationships, communities, technology, and nature. Equally, our internal systems are connected as well through physical and communicative means. Our bodies are literally connected via ligaments, muscles, bones, and cells. In addition, there are pathways and channels of communication within our body that "talk" to one another. Typically, communication occurs within the body through chemical or electric means. Most of the time, both forms of communication are involved on some level. Understanding these connections and forms of communication can help us understand our bodies and how we relate to the outside world.

As the title of the chapter suggests, we (both men and women) experience thoughts and emotions. The title is a play on words based on the book title *As a Man Thinketh* by James Allen. I remember reading this book as a young man and feeling enlightened by the idea that our thoughts impact who we are. James Allen believed that how we think impacts what we do and leads to who we become. If a person thinks it, it can happen. However, research suggests that thoughts alone don't seem to make up the entire story of what impacts our internal communications relating to wellness. They are just one piece of the pie.

When I was in graduate school, I remember learning about different mechanisms of change, and scientists continue to study what factors influence our willingness to make changes in our lives. If someone wants to lose weight or improve their eating habits or progress in a relationship, what change is most important? Is it the way we think, or how we feel? Is it the actions we take? Do we have to have certain thoughts first to act in certain ways? Or do we have to feel something in order to act? Do our actions lead to new thoughts?

When scientists research and discover answers to these questions, they usually develop a theories. There are a wide range of theories for what makes us tick. Some believe that changing our thoughts is what makes the difference (cognitivists); others believe that changing behaviors or actions will lead to thought change (behavioralists), while others believe it is a combination of both (cognitive-behavioralists). Another group of scientists believe that emotions are extremely important to the change process as well. You will find approaches that combine emotions and thoughts (rational-emotive approaches), approaches that combine emotions and relational patterns (attachment-based theories or emotionally focused approaches). As mentioned in chapter 2, some take a systemic approach or relational and patterned approach in which the focus is on how thoughts, behaviors, and emotions are integrated into our connections within ourselves, with others, and with the world.

So, which one is right? Do we have evidence that any of these factors seem to make the *most* difference? I think if you would ask most social scientists, they would say that certain parts of the debate are over. Similar to the nature versus nurture debate (do our genetics or our experience impact how we act the most?), the question isn't which one is right anymore. In the nature versus nurture debate, scientists know that both genes and our environment impact us on a deep level. The question now is how much of each affects each behavior. In other words, we know that certain conditions are highly genetic (alcoholism, schizophrenia, and some chronic illnesses); yet even these conditions suggest that an environmental factor is still at play. The genetic tendency seems to be turned on by events and actions that take place in our lives. Other conditions seem to have a genetic tendency with a much higher environmental influence (obesity, type 2 diabetes, depression, and so on). Thus, both nature and nurture impact our lives. Equally, thoughts, emotions, behaviors and relational patterns all impact our ability to change. The question isn't "Which one is most important?" The question now is "How do we integrate all these elements to help people live well?" They are all important because they each play a part in our lives.

I have found that there is a wide range of doors and windows that can be used to get inside the change process. Some people will say they have tried everything when attempting to make a change. However, I have found that usually what is occurring is that person is trying to open the same door over and over again and it continues to remain shut. The answer is to try multiple doors, which could include thought pathways, behavior pathways, emotional pathways and even relational pathways. You never know which one might be open. Let me give you a few examples.

I remember working with a couple that said they were on the verge of divorce. The gentleman was a successful CFO for a large company and the wife was a talented journalist. I had recently been having a lot of success working with couples using emotional pathways, and the research suggested that most couples do better quicker through an emotional intervention. Out of habit, I went with the same route with this couple. I began to ask about their patterns of behavior and the emotional hurt behind them. I discovered both would distance themselves from one another in times of stress and that the wife felt alone. The husband had a difficult time expressing any emotion. After hitting a brick wall for a couple of weeks with the couple (trying to open that same door over and over again), I decided to go a cognitive route. I got into an analytical conversation with the husband about some theories he had been reading about psychology. I quickly discovered that he would light up when we had engaging, intellectual conversation. Surprisingly, the wife seemed to light up as well. After some more assessment, I found out that the son had been diagnosed with autism and the parents' families had a history of what used to be called Asperger's syndrome (now an autistic spectrum disorder). Long story short, people with autism typically have a difficult time fully processing emotion. The connection this couple needed was actually at a cognitive and behavioral level. Once they understood that their distance was related to a lack of time spent with one another on areas that helped them connect and that past hurts could be resolved by sharing their concerns with one another, the couple connected quickly. In all honesty, it was the quickest turnaround I have ever seen in a couple, and I originally was going through the "wrong" door. This couple thrived on change through thoughts that led to emotional and relational connection.

How can this example relate to you? Some of you may be trying to think yourself into making a healthy change. Others may be trying to set goal after goal (behaviors) in order to make those changes. Others may be waiting to feel a certain way before they engage in certain changes, while others may be trying to change patterns of a relationship in order to gain more support to engage in change. None of these approaches are wrong. However, if you have tried a certain approach over and over, it is like trying to open that closed door that is bolted shut for whatever reason. Try another door. This doesn't mean try a different solution; rather, try a different type of solution.

The purpose of this chapter is to give you more insight on how to take advantage of the amazing mental and emotional components of your brain and body. In addition, I would like to touch upon how your thoughts and emotions impact the various components of your life.

WHAT ARE THOUGHTS?

Some of us may imagine thoughts as "mysterious clouds" in our brain that float around in some random manner. I don't know if most of us imagine thoughts as cells engaging in electrical and chemical exchanges with one another. I don't want to get too technical here, but it would be good to cover a few basic ideas behind how our brain and body works together. Inside our brains, there are different types of cells, including neurons. Neurons are elongated cells that have tentacle-like arms on two sides of the cell (one end for receiving messages and one end for sending messages). On one end, these tentacles receive chemicals (neurotransmitters) from another cell. The neuron receives the chemical message and converts it into an electrical impulse that will be sent down the cell like an electrical wire, which will then tell the cell to release more chemicals. There are millions of neurons creating pathways throughout the brain similar to a series of wires going through our brain.

Some of these neurotransmitters in our brain can impact our mood, motivation, and ability to focus, as well as other functions in our body. For example, you may have heard of an SSRI (selective serotonin reuptake inhibitor). Usually, SSRI medications are used for depression or anxiety. Serotonin is a chemical that impacts our mood; if we have more serotonin released, we usually feel more content. Serotonin is one of the neurotransmitters that neurons release. The tentacles on the neuron will often suck up extra neurotransmitters that are released kind of like a vacuum. A reuptake inhibitor basically allows the serotonin to be out and about for longer by blocking the vacuum, which, in turn, helps us feel better and have more energy.

Another neurotransmitter that seems to be important for motivation and enjoying certain activities is called dopamine. Dopamine is sometimes called the reward neurotransmitter because it is released when we begin to associate a certain thought or behavior with obtaining something in return. Unfortunately, this can lead to negative associations as well, including addictions to drugs, alcohol, sex, and really anything.

At this point we know that thoughts are partially tied to long strings of neurons that form pathways in our brain. We also know that these neurons release chemicals in our brain that impact how we feel, our motivation, and our ability to focus as well, as other mechanisms. An important point to make here is that these pathways can change; they aren't set in stone. I often like to use the example of walking in a forest. The first time you walk in a forest

— with no set path, you may have a difficult time because you have to clear away brush, move limbs, and fight through the natural growth of the forest. However, if you kept walking that same route, eventually a path would form. Equally, if you stopped walking the path, the forest would cover the path with new growth. The pathways in our brain work the same way. There is a concept called Hebb's learning rule that basically says that if we keep thinking a certain thought or set of thoughts, that pathway invites other neurons over and makes the pathway stronger. It becomes easier to think that way. Equally, if we place barriers or engage in other ways of thinking instead of going down the same path, the neurons eventually leave, and there is no pathway. What does this mean? The way we think and keep thinking or not thinking literally changes the physical makeup of our brain! In other words, phrases like "That is just who I am" or "That is the way I am made" don't always accurately reflect our ability to change the way we think. We can literally change who we are by thinking differently.

In summary, thoughts are a combination of electrical and chemical messages that communicate with our body. Neurons in our brain form pathways based on how we think, act, and relate with the world. These pathways can be strengthened, weakened, or even removed based on how often we think along those pathways. In other words, we can change the pathways.

WHAT CAN WE DO WITH OUR THOUGHTS?

It is important to note that even though James Allen, in his book *As a Man Thinketh,* was not completely accurate about the influence of thought (he wrote it in 1903—he was ahead of his time!), many of the concepts in his book are still relevant today. In many ways, our thoughts impact who we are, how we react, how we see the world, how we interact with others, how we handle pain and joy, how we feel, and even how our body responds to outside stimuli. Our thoughts are very powerful.

There are many concepts related to positive thinking and how to overcome barriers in our thought processes. Throughout the years and after working with thousands of clients, I would like to cover some of the more common principles that I have found helpful with myself and my clients:

1. Know what you can and can't control.

This is by far the most difficult and most beneficial thought process that could use a little changing in each of us. Most of us have worries and stressors that are on our minds constantly. We will learn more about stress in chapter 15, but I would like to note that stress is actually not the issue. It is how we think about stress or anxiety. When we look at what we actually worry about, we find that only a small percentage of our worries are actually in our control. Here are a few examples: the past (can't change it), the economy (wish we could do something about it), the weather (would be nice to control), or how others react (we can influence others, but they have their choice).

For other worries, we may have some amount of control but not in this very moment. For example, I may be thinking about that exam or deadline tomorrow; I may be thinking about cleaning the house or running errands; I may be thinking about what will happen this year in my business or career. In reality, most of these worries are quite healthy and help us keep ourselves organized. However, we don't have to worry about them in moments that don't matter. People who are able to master this skill actually schedule times to worry. For example, I will worry about my deadline or exam when I am studying for the exam or working on the deadline; other times, I won't because I know I have a time scheduled to worry about it. I will worry about cleaning my house when I am engaged in cleaning my house at a set time. You will learn more about a concept called mindfulness in chapter 6. Mindfulness is the ability to stay in the present and focus on what is useful and important in that moment. Mindfulness often brings peace of mind and more life enjoyment. In summary, when you know when to let go of those things you can't control, worry about those things in their proper time, and enjoy the moment, your thoughts let you see the world and your place in it.

When I was a young father, I was always worrying about school, work, money, and other decisions and would get caught up and distracted by my worries. I would be playing at the park with my two-year-old daughter and be present physically but not mentally. I was going through the motions, but I wouldn't be savoring the moment. I wasn't noticing the flower she picked for me along with the smile that came with young innocence. I wish I had those moments back. If I had a chance to talk to myself back then as a young father, I would say to myself, "Jared, things will work out. There will be ups and downs, but you will get through them all. There will always be work, deadlines, challenges, and so on; you will only have your daughter or son once. You will never experience them at two years old again. When they turn three, it is gone. Enjoy the moments. Those moments are more important." I made a commitment to myself a long time ago that when I play with my kids, I will play with my kids and let other worries go away for a moment. I still struggle with this at times, but over the years I have learned to savor the special moments more and more.

2. Know when to say yes and know when to say no.

This skill is related to our thoughts and other people. There are a couple of chapters related to how we interact with others, so I won't go into too many details at this point. However, it is important to know how to mentally understand boundary setting. Some of us say yes way too often. If anyone asks anything of us, we do it. This can create burnout both mentally and physically. Saying yes too much usually is related to the belief that by saying yes, we will be more liked or more accepted. However, if you can train yourself to say yes only when it is related to the following areas, you are more likely to use this skill to connect and progress at a high level: (a) say yes to requests that you have time for and will enjoy; (b) say yes to requests that are using your special skills and talents and fit your life goals (more on this later); and (c) say yes to requests that help you meet the everyday demands and chores of life when they are fairly distributed amongst others involved. (This means you can ask your spouse to help with the dishes or the lawn.)

[handwritten margin note: When to say yes.]

3. Focus on what we want and what is right more than what is wrong.

There are so many books and strategies out there on a positive thinking and improving our mood. I personally enjoy the following:

- *As a Man Thinketh* by James Allen
- *The Greatest Salesman in the World* by Og Mandino
- *Feeling Good* by David Burns
- *Happiness: Unlocking the Mysteries of Psychological Wealth* by Ed Diener and Robert Biswas-Diener
- *The Anatomy of Peace* by The Arbinger Institute

Most of these books tend to have a common theme, which is to focus more on what we want out of life and what is going well than to focus on what is wrong. I'm not suggesting you never consider what is wrong; however, most of us are much better at explaining what is wrong with our lives than explaining what we would like life to be. There are a few techniques from an approach called Solution-Focused Therapy that can help us shift our thinking. The most common technique used in this approach is called "the miracle question." The miracle question uses the following scenario:

Pretend that in the middle of the night a miracle happened and you wake up in the morning and your life is where you would like it to be. What would it look like? How would you know the miracle happened? How would you be spending your time? What would you be doing? What would you not be doing?

The miracle question is designed to get you in the mode of thinking how you would like life to be. You can't say you would win the lottery or find a genie and get three wishes or anything like that. However, you get the chance to consider how you could realistically have a life that is within your reach. Some of the questions that come after your response include, "What is preventing you from getting there?" "Are there some small steps that will help you move in that direction?" In general, focusing on what is right or how you would like life to be will actually create pathways in our brain that will more likely lead us to those places in the future.

[margin note: Solution focused miracle question]

4. Learn from the past, live in the present, plan for the future.

We learned from the first suggestion that we can't change the past, but we can learn from it and then let it go. We learned from suggestion 3 that we can use positive thinking to consider our future and make steps to reach the future. We also learned from suggestion 1 that when we can focus on the present through mindfulness techniques and enjoying the moment, we can enjoy the simple treasures of life. I have met people who live in the past too much and experience "the Uncle Rico" syndrome. If you have seen the film *Napoleon Dynamite*, you'll remember that Uncle Rico buys a time machine from a catalog to go back in time so he can change his play on the football field and win state. During the entire movie, he is focusing on the "what-if" scenarios of his past. *If only he could go back and make a few changes to his play on the field, life would be so much better now! He would be in the NFL, with lots of money—happy!* We don't want to fall into the same trap of thinking about how life could be different "if only." Equally, I have met people who live too much in the future: "Life will be better when I am finished with school, get a new job, or little Johnny starts school." They forget to enjoy where they are today; they forget to enjoy the journey. We don't want to fall into the trap of denying ourselves happiness by thinking it will only come in the future. We can always plan for the future to help us understand the journey to take; however, planning for the future is different than living in the future. In the end, we can learn from the past, live in the present, and plan for the future.

ARE THERE THOUGHTS THAT GET IN THE WAY?

Most people will experience some form of depression or anxiety in their life. Some will experience bouts of feeling depressed more severely. We discussed that some medications can help people experience a temporary boost in serotonin or other neurotransmitters to be able to focus better, have more energy, or have more motivation. However, research suggests that a combination of addressing negative thoughts and behaviors along with boosts of neurotransmitters has the most effective, long-term outcomes. First and foremost, I want to share with you some of the most common ways to naturally boost neurotransmitters like serotonin. (I'm not necessarily against medications but feel that we can all learn how to naturally access our body's healing abilities.)

- Walk at least thirty minutes per day or engage in more cardio.
- Get outside in the sunlight.
- Engage in hobbies you enjoy.
- Get enough sleep (seven to eight hours, preferably).
- Connect with others socially.
- Pray or meditate.
- Connect with nature and/or animals.
- Engage in touch, affection, and sexual intimacy with a committed partner.
- Reduce processed foods and caffeine and eliminate smoking.

When we naturally boost neurotransmitters like serotonin, changing our thoughts becomes easier. Actually, when you engage in these activities more, you are changing those pathways, which results changing your thoughts! We sometimes call negative thought patterns defense mechanisms or irrational beliefs. Defense mechanisms are ways we react to seemingly negative experiences or beliefs. For example, we may rationalize behaviors ("I drink too much so I won't use drugs"); project, which means getting upset with a trait someone else displays that we wish to deny in ourselves (blaming the kids for not measuring up because your boss yelled at you that day); or be in denial.

Irrational beliefs are belief systems that put us in a frame of mind that make it impossible for us to succeed or progress. For example, teenagers will often believe that they are the only one that is experiencing what they are experiencing or that everyone is noticing them and their imperfections. (These are normal teenage irrational beliefs, by the way; even though they are irritating, teens typically grow out of them. Yeah!) Adults have many irrational beliefs as well: "I can't change," "Bad things always happen to me," or "People never understand me." Usually, irrational beliefs have an "all or nothing" feel to them. "Always" and "never" statements typically fall into this line of thinking.

Being aware of your thoughts and how you think will automatically begin to change pathways. Today, we know that it typically takes at least thirty days of intense "different thinking" to engage in a change process in your brain. The most difficult types of behaviors reinforced by poor thinking (for example, alcoholism) might take about a year of different thinking and behaviors. In fact, that is why the one-year sobriety award is so important in Alcoholics Anonymous (AA); we didn't know it at the time due to a lack of brain imaging technology, but a significant change in the brain seems to occur after one year. The brain normalizes. What an amazing body we have to be able to change so quickly and significantly! The more I have learned about the brain, the more hope I have that our bodies and brains have the tools to help us meet almost any challenge. Our thoughts are a significant tool we can access for that change. *The brain completely normalizes after one year.*

Small habits = 30 days   Huge habits = 1 year

✳ WHAT ARE EMOTIONS?

Emotions are complex reactions to mechanisms in our body that stem from thoughts in our brain, neurotransmitters released that impact our brain, and neuropeptides that are released in the hypothalamus (also in the brain) that flow throughout our body and communicate with different systems in our body. *emotions* For example, if I am thinking something negative and am experiencing a common thought process of hopelessness, my hypothalamus will release neuropeptides that match my emotional state. These neuropeptides will tell my muscles and joints to ache more, will tell my digestive system to inflame, and will tell my body that I am tired and need to maintain energy leading to feeling lethargic. Each emotional state is based on these neuropeptides that are released based on thoughts and behaviors.

We do know that some of the most powerful emotional states are created when we involve other people through experiences. For example, have you ever overcome a difficult challenge or shared in a common endeavor with others and felt a stronger bond with them afterward? Have you developed a more intimate relationship with someone due to being vulnerable and sharing your emotional state with them? It is likely you have experienced the intensity of emotion with others. We will discuss these emotional concepts in the context of relationships more in chapter 12. For now, it is important to note that emotions often provide a sense of bonding, purpose, and motivation as we engage in certain thoughts and behaviors with ourselves and others.

The neuropeptides that influence our emotional state in each cell in our body have receptors that receive information from these neuropeptides. These receptors are like keyholes and the neuropeptides are like keys telling the cell to do something. Thus, we may have a rapid heart rate when we feel scared or achy joints when we feel depressed. The most amazing thing happens with some of these cells when they get bombarded with the usual neuropeptides. When the cell splits, the cell will have more receptors (keyholes) for the common neuropeptides and less holes for the less common ones. What does this mean? If we keep thinking in a manner that leads to depressive moods, our cells over time will become used to this state and make it easier for the body to feel this way. Equally, it will make it more difficult to feel other ways because there are less receptors (keyholes) for the other emotional states. In other words, the way we think, behave, and relate with others leads to the release of certain emotional states that lead our cells to change and become that emotional state. How we think and feel changes our body—literally! Our cells change over time based on what we give them. They adapt to maintain a homeostasis, as discussed in chapter 2. When I learned this, I felt empowered. I don't have to be the current body or person if I don't want to. I can literally change the makeup of my cells through how I think, feel, and relate with others. I am tempted to go into more details about how emotional states lead to one of the most important survival mechanisms we have—attachment. It's even stronger than food and water based on some awful studies in the past where baby monkeys or rats would starve themselves when they were given the choice between a bond with a mother figure or food. Chapter 12 will go in more detail on this. It is important to realize though that the experiences we have combined with our emotional states may be one of the most powerful forces of change we have.

WHAT ABOUT DEPRESSION AND ANXIETY?

We know that depression and anxiety for most people stems from a combination of physical factors in the brain and environmental factors that include our relationships, physical health, nutrition, work, peers, fitness, ways we think, and how we balance our lives. The concepts in this book are actually designed to help someone with depression and anxiety in addition to other areas. We do know that for most individuals, depression or anxiety will be temporary. We also know that most people will experience some level of depression and anxiety throughout their lives. This is especially true following significant difficult events like a trauma, unexpected death, chronic illness, or divorce. Some people believe that they are feeling depressed or anxious because of something they did wrong. They feel guilty or embarrassed or weak about the symptoms of depression or anxiety that they are experiencing. Although some decisions can lead someone to feel depressed or anxious, many of us experience depression and anxiety as a part of the challenges of life and in part due to chemical factors in our brain. We need to remember that our brain is an organ just like our heart, lungs, or liver. Just as our heart, lungs and liver can have disease, our brain can experience disease or dysfunction that mainly occurs through chemicals we already discussed called neurotransmitters. Fortunately, just as our heart and lungs can heal, our brain can heal as well.

Although we know how to identify depression and anxiety better today, we aren't always completely sure when the depression or anxiety is more related to chemical dysfunction or lifestyle patterns. Thus, we tend to treat both areas and adjust from there. It is always important to consult a professional when considering how to handle depression, anxiety, or other mental health concerns. In general, I recommend the following to clients or patients I have worked with:

1. Increase levels of cardio (walking thirty minutes per day increases serotonin, which decreases depression).

2. Get outside more (being in nature and having more exposure to sunlight has shown to decrease symptoms).

3. Connect with loved ones (talking with a spouse, friend, or family member often has been shown to both decrease symptoms and protect you from more symptoms).

4. Healthy eating (eating more fruits and vegetables and less sugars and caffeinated beverages)

5. Engage in hobbies (many don't feel like engaging in hobbies; however, many report once they start they feel better).

6. Prioritize and organize your life (having more life balance and ways to cope with stress).

[handwritten margin note: Reduces anxiety + depression]

Many of these areas will be discussed in more detail throughout the book. It is important to note that engaging in these behaviors will not always "cure" someone from depression or anxiety. However, the symptoms reduce for many people, and when combined with professional treatment when needed, success rates increase even more.

CAN OUR WORDS AND LANGUAGE IMPACT OUR THOUGHTS AND EMOTIONS?

Yes. That is the simple answer. In fact, most of our thoughts are formed by developing language. We do know there are universal forms of communication that supersede language (tears, smiles, and so on). However, most of our concepts of the world and how we think are based on our experience with others and the formation of language. There are several major theories that exist that suggest one mode of change is paying more attention to the stories we have about ourselves and the world. Trying to change negative thought patterns can be abstract for many of us. You may be racking your brain, considering what negative thought patterns you have. It is easier to consider the stories we have about our lives. We do know that all cultures have storytelling traditions. Even today, we tell stories through plays, books, movies, poems, blogs, tweets, and Facebook posts.

What is your story? What character do you play? What chapters have been written, and what is coming next? The words and ways you talk about your story will give you insight into how you see yourself and the world. Some of you may not be fully aware of your story and will begin to realize that as you verbalize your story you will discover certain beliefs and expectations you have placed in your life that make it difficult for you to progress. Some people define their whole lives off of a certain event that happened in the past. The Uncle Rico syndrome from Napoleon Dynamite comes to mind again. Uncle Rico is always trying to re-live his high school years as a quarterback and even buys that mail-order time machine to go back and have one more chance to make the big play! Have you made a mistake that you can't let go of and your story seems to always be linked to that mistake? Redefining your story can be healing, and using a professional can be helpful in this process at times. Some common techniques used to help develop your story are illustrated in the following example:

I was working with a gentleman from Mississippi who was court-ordered to inpatient treatment for crystal meth addiction. He was weathered, malnourished and lost. He had two teardrop tattoos next to his eyes. Being the naïve young professional at the time, I didn't know what the teardrop tattoos meant. He explained that each teardrop was for a murder he had committed. These murders defined his life as he was going to spend most of his life in prison.

He was a quiet, shamed man and couldn't look me in the eye. I asked to him to tell me his story. As he did, I picked out places to expand his story. He expanded on times that he made his dad proud or did something great in school. He discussed how others in his family suffered from drugs and he suffered himself. He began to realize that his life wasn't defined by this one act of murdering two individuals; his life was a full tapestry of good times, proud moments, suffering with others and suffering himself. He began to stop placing a magnifying glass on his mistake and take a different role in his story of life. I asked him to name his biggest challenge and use descriptive words to help illustrate it. He called his shame and guilt of making mistakes "ugly tar." It stuck on him and he couldn't get it off; it slowed him down and was always on his mind. I asked him if there were times that he was able to get the "ugly tar" off? He said when he was helping someone else, the ugly tar seemed to go away. "I don't want them to experience that same ugly tar," he says. "I especially like giving hope and praise to younger men because I didn't get much of it myself." I wasn't able to see him much more than a month. I do remember one of the last times I saw him—he smiled and looked me in the eye for a brief moment and had a slight twinkle in his eye. Then he quickly lowered his head.

Looking back, I wish I would have given him a hug and told him he had goodness in him. Mistakes of a young professional. I learned a lot about stories from him. More than anything, I learned that we don't fully realize how the small good moments that we give to others can be lifelines for some in the future. I doubt the teacher that gave this man a compliment as a little boy had any idea that he would hold onto that thought in future years to stay connected to hope. I also learned that we can redefine our lives at any time. There are many chapters left to write in our book of life. We can always edit past chapters as well based on how we see it in the context of the bigger picture. This man left with a feeling that his new mission in life was to serve others as best as he could in the situation given.

ACTION ITEMS

As you consider how your thoughts, emotions, and stories impact your life, consider some of the following action items:

1. Choose one area of improvement regarding the way you see life. Some examples include:

- Consider saying yes or no in a more balanced manner.
- Let go of the past more.
- Don't live in the future too much ("the grass is greener on the other side" syndrome).
- Enjoy the moments more in the present.
- Focus more on what you want in life or what is right.
- Take charge of your own happiness.
- Enjoy the journey more than the destination.

2. Consider writing or telling your story.

Some people use a journal or blog to do this. Others may just begin to share this with people they trust, including family members, a spouse, or even a professional helper.

3. Consider engaging in activities that increase serotonin naturally.

Such activities include walking at least thirty minutes per day or engaging in more cardio; getting outside in the sunlight; engaging in hobbies you enjoy; getting enough sleep (seven to eight hours preferably); connecting with others socially; engaging in prayer or meditation; connecting with nature and/or animals; engaging in touch, affection, and sexual intimacy with committed partners; reducing processed foods and caffeine; and eliminating smoking.

CONCLUSION

It is important to recognize that our thoughts and emotions are tied to our physical bodies and relationships. They are tied to how we interact with others in our families, careers, and communities. When I was a young kid, I remember thinking I was built a certain way and couldn't change. I was extremely shy—so shy that I'm pretty sure a lot of people thought something was wrong with me. I was also a sensitive kid that would get embarrassed a lot and would cry. The other day I listened to my son Kai (four years old) crying in the other room saying, "What is wrong with me? Why can't I stop crying?!" I'm sure I felt the same many times but didn't have the insight at the time to voice it. Today, I'm still shy but now enjoy traveling around the world meeting different people and cultures. I actually make it a point to get to know the locals and live like the locals do. As a child, I would have been too hesitant to get to know a new person, let alone visit a new country. I changed how I perceived people by realizing each person has a story to share and something to teach me. I still get hesitant when I first meet people but I am a different person now. I have new thoughts and emotions about myself. I continue to work on them. I have hope that I can continue to create pathways that will lead me to higher ways of thinking and being. I feel the same about you.

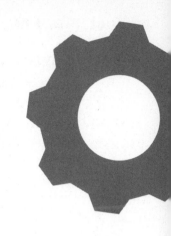

4 CHANGE

FINDING OUR TRUE MOTIVATION

BY MICHAEL OLSON, PHD, &
CATALINA TRIANA, MD

"TRANSFORMATION IS A PROCESS, NOT AN EVENT."[1]
—JOHN P. KOTTER

MICHAEL M. OLSON, PHD, *is an associate professor and director of behavioral medicine at the University of Texas Medical Branch (UTMB). He earned a master's degree in marriage and family therapy (MFT) from Brigham Young University and a PhD in MFT from Kansas State University with post-doctoral training in Behavioral Medicine from UTMB. He is a member of the Motivational Interviewing Network of Trainers (MINT). He is passionate about integration of behavioral health into the patient-centered medical home (PCMH) and the future of family medicine.*

CATALINA TRIANA, MD, *is the associate program director of the John Muir/UCSF Family Medicine Residency in Walnut Creek, California—a new residency program with focus on patient engagement and interprofessional team care for the underserved. She received her medical degree from the Universidad Javeriana in Bogotá, Colombia. She completed her residency training and a two-year family systems fellowship at UTMB in Galveston, Texas. She has been teaching behavioral medicine, patient-centered communication, and primary care counseling skills to family medicine residents and medical students since 2002. Dr. Triana is a motivational interviewing trainer (member of MINT) and is passionate about teaching skills to facilitate health behavior change.*

Editor's note: Mike and Catalina see thousands of patients every year come through the family medicine clinic. They are in the trenches, dealing with families in crisis on an almost daily basis—and they see what works and what doesn't. Over the years, they have navigated this difficult terrain of helping people with their health and wellness by developing models that impact change more effectively. Both have been instrumental in developing the overall WholeFIT approach. Their approach to motivation has been recognized nationally and globally.

INTRODUCTION

A young mother came to the emergency department of a small community hospital. She arrived with multiple head injuries and cuts to her arms. Once imaging was completed, I discovered that she had sustained multiple bone fractures after being assaulted by her husband. As I met and discussed the situation with her, she determined not to call the police or press charges for the assault. She insisted that her husband was a "good man" and would never hurt their child, and the only reason he had hurt her was because she had made him angry. She did, however, agree to see me in my outpatient clinic a week later. I met with her off and on as she continued in an abusive relationship, not willing or ready to make a change. This continued until she returned one day with a determination that I had not seen in her to that point. I asked what had happened and she reported that she and her husband and had been in a fight and he had thrown an object toward her and missed. The object instead crashed into their young child. She immediately picked up their child, left, and found shelter. She explained that seeing their child harmed that way had made something "click" inside her that sparked the resolve to leave and never return to this abusive man. She had come into my clinic to get help with the steps she would need to make this long-awaited and needed change.

Once the line was crossed—once his abuse impacted their child's wellbeing and not just hers—she found the motivation she needed to seek a change. Up until then, her belief system had allowed for his abusive acts toward herself, but when his abuse harmed their child, she found the will to save herself through her child.

Often, as a result of maligned choices, we find ourselves spiritually, physically, emotionally, relationally, or psychologically "over the line" and ready to make a change. The challenge is to raise this discrepancy and cognitive dissonance without waiting for life or circumstances to raise it for us—sometimes with dire consequences. The purpose of this chapter is to help you understand and impact your own levels of motivation.

Change does not often happen instantaneously, nor does it occur in a vacuum. Change is a process and often happens in the context of our closest social relationships. We affect others by the changes we make in our lives and are affected by the changes others are making as well. Like touching one part of a wind chime and seeing the rest of the chime move in concert, so it is with change. How does change come about, and what will predict change happening and continuing to happen in our lives?

I. MOTIVATION AND CHANGE

Heraclitus, the pre-Socratic Greek philosopher, is often attributed to saying, "The only thing that is constant is change."[3] Most of us are engaged in some state or process of change (physical, emotional, psychological, relational, spiritual, etc.) throughout our lives. We are often in some state of consolidating change, contemplating change, or actively experimenting with steps and changes. Browse the local library or the bestseller list online and you will discover a multitude of books, articles, blogs, studies, and so on that focus on change, in all its forms.

The center or core of what we know about the change process has to do with *motivation*. It is true that there are many sources and types of motivation, benevolent and otherwise; however, the motivation that has been shown to yield the most power to catalyze change is *intrinsic* and springs from one's own core beliefs and values. Thus, the goal is to help you understand how to find your own intrinsic motivation and identify the steps that will help you start and continue your personal journey toward health and wellness.

Key Principles of Motivation and Change

Stages of Change: Thinking about Change as a Process

One helpful way of thinking about how change occurs was developed by researchers James Prochaska and Carlo DiClemente[4] and is based on their research in addictions. They found that change often happens in stages. Their "stages of change model" include (1) precontemplation, (2) contemplation, (3) preparation, (3) action, (4) maintenance, and (5) relapse. Each of these stages will be briefly discussed.

- *Precontemplation*: Change is not part of the agenda. "My weight is not an issue."

- *Contemplation*: The contemplator is weighing out the pros and cons, or thinking about the reasons for being concerned or not concerned, motivated or not motivated to make a change. Most of us find ourselves in this state of wanting to change but not wanting to change—a feeling of ambivalence. "I'd love to lose weight, I just don't have the will to stick to a diet."

- *Preparation*: Prochaska and DiClemente found that there is often a seminal event or fulcrum that tips the balance forward in a person's life. This balance can shift for any number of reasons and seems to always be personal.

In the years of my working at various hospitals, I have had conversations with patients at moments when things seem to be darkest, and I will hear things like, "I've got to do something about this problem!" or "If I don't figure this out once and for all, I will lose everything I care about." These types of declarative statements can often open a window for a patient to move from the contemplation stage to the preparation stage.

- *Action*: When people make a decision to take steps forward and change something about their life, they enter the action stage. Those who embark in "action" actively and intentionally work toward the goal of change. This may happen with or without any professional assistance. If we seriously reflect on our own efforts to make changes in our lives (New Year's Resolutions, for example), we will freely admit that the process of starting a change and the process of continuing a change are often very different propositions.

- *Maintenance*: Those who continue with making changes for six months are considered moving into the maintenance stage of change, where the concerns shift toward recognizing what will be needed to continue change successfully and anticipate threats to derailing one's efforts. This stage may last up to five years but of course varies based on individual self-efficacy and the nature of the problem or area of change.

- *Relapse*: Those who are able to integrate these changes in their lives are able to make a permanent exit from these stages, while those who "slip" or "relapse" find their way back through the steps of contemplation, determination, and action, depending on their readiness to keep moving forward.

Relapse isn't failure. It's part of the change process. A very helpful contribution from the stages of change research is the understanding that slips (minor setbacks) and relapses (major setbacks) are a normal part of the change process and are to be expected. The data suggests that it takes on average four to seven times through the stages of change wheel before most people are able to stay with changes long term. Often we embark on the change process from a dichotomous or black-and-white mind-set: "Either I change or I don't"; "I'm successful at this or I'm a failure"; or "I've not eaten cake for two months, but because I had a slice today, I've blown it and my efforts are useless." If slips and relapses are an expected part of the change process, we are better able to think about change on a continuum with questions like "What did I learn about myself or my situation from this slip or relapse?" and "What will I need to do differently or anticipate as a barrier the next time I approach this situation?" The goal here is to restart the effort, being better prepared to be more successful the next time around.

II. VALUE SORTING: BUILDING DISCREPANCY BETWEEN VALUES AND BEHAVIOR

With the backdrop of the stages of change in mind, the next and most critical principle for mobilizing our internal motivation includes looking carefully at what our deepest values and beliefs are. *What is it you care most deeply about? What are the things you know are true or most important and contribute to your sense of meaning and purpose in life? What do you want your health for?* Ironically, it is often in the darkest moments when our decisions or the decisions of others threaten these most cherished values and beliefs that change can spark and take hold.

When values and beliefs become "out of sync" or incongruent with our behaviors or with what is happening in our lives, the typical result is a cognitive dissonance or internal friction that can often build discrepancy and motivation for change to live more consistent with our beliefs and values.

Examples

1. A young adult may consider cutting back on his smoking if his cough affects his ability to play soccer with his buddies. (Behavior: smoking. Values in conflict: exercise and friendship.)

2. A grandmother may be more likely to quit drinking if it means she gets to see her grandchildren. (Behavior: drinking. Value in conflict: family.)

3. Staying on a diet is easier if you have a high school reunion coming up. (Behavior: diet. Value in conflict: pride.)

III. IMPORTANCE: SCALING CHANGE THROUGH MOTIVATIONAL INTERVIEWING

One of the main contributions of this work is to dispel the idea that change is an event rather than a process. Here are some ideas we use when helping clients try to begin the process of making positive changes in their lives. We start by teaching them that change usually doesn't happen overnight as a single decision. Rather, it's a process. One method we use is to help clients to scale the importance of a change they are contemplating by giving it a number. A zero means the change is "not at all important" and a ten means it is "extremely important."

The idea of scaling (or measuring) importance (and later confidence) comes from the work of psychologists Miller and Rollnick,[5] who have studied and written extensively on the process of change from a clinical perspective. They have articulated an approach called *motivational interviewing*, or MI. Here's how it works:

Let's take the example of someone with diabetes. Taking care of a chronic disease like diabetes requires self-discipline and determination. A person with uncontrolled diabetes has to check his or her blood sugars, follow a diet, and take or inject medications twice—sometimes three times day. Without having any uncomfortable symptoms, it is hard to stay motivated to do this day in and day out. As a physician I could simply tell the patient all the important reasons to take care of the diabetes to avoid complications, but if I am concerned with helping that particular patient find the motivation to control the diabetes, it would be helpful for me to have some idea how likely it is for the patient to actually do what I've recommended. In order to assess a patient's willingness to make a change in behavior that will be required to protect future health, I could ask, "How important, on a scale from zero to ten, is it for you to keep your sugars under control?" The patient's response would help me assess readiness, and as I explore it further would give me insight into the values that may guide his or her behavior. Imagine that the patient says, "Doc, it is about a five—not unimportant but not the most important thing." Next, I will ask a question the patient might not expect: "What makes it the number it is and not a lower number? What makes it a five and not a three or a four?" There is often a number lower than the number a patient gives me, even if it is a one.

I ask these questions because I'm trying to discover reasons for change or values that make taking diabetes meds and testing blood sugar at least minimally important. Once I understand this, I'll have some insight as to what might need to happen to convince a patient to be more careful and concerned about treating his or her diabetes.

When a patient considers why the answer was five and not a three or a four, he or she might say, "I've heard that uncontrolled diabetes may lead to blindness. I am an artist and I cannot let that happen. I have to preserve my vision." Now that the patient has identified why maintaining good vision is important, it will be easier to help him or her find the motivation to make necessary diabetes treatment a priority so good vision can be preserved.

Again, it is often the course of life events and circumstances that raises importance for us (a diagnosis of a chronic illness, the loss of a limb, separation from loved ones, and so on) by revealing our underlying values or the awareness of what matters most. The challenge is for us to do the mental work necessary to raise importance to a level that helps us determine to initiate a change in our lives.

IV. CONFIDENCE: SCALING OUR STEPS FORWARD TO INCREASE CONFIDENCE

Once importance has been raised and established and the reasons for change are clear (the patient and I have identified core values and beliefs), the next step is to scale (measure) the patient's confidence. Using the same scale (0 = not at all confident, 10 = extremely confident), I ask, "How confident do you feel that you can make a change in this area of your life?"

A colleague said something years ago at a conference I attended that has stayed with me since: "You only do what you feel confident doing." Most people want to feel capable and effective in the things they try and tend to avoid or delay things where there is a high risk of failure. In scaling confidence, most people will not choose a zero, even if confidence is very low. If a patient says her confidence in her ability to walk at least a mile a day is only a four, the next question to be asked is, "Why a four and not a lower number?" This question is meant to evoke or elicit the confidence that *does* exist and to understand it. Breaking this idea down a bit further, we might continue with the example of someone with diabetes.

Q: "How confident do you feel you could lower your blood sugars?"

A: "About a four."

Q: "What makes it a four and not a two or a three?"

A: "I was able to control my blood sugars when I was first diagnosed. I kept a diet and a blood sugar diary, but that was years ago."

Q: "What would have to happen for your confidence number to be a little higher? Say, a 5 or a 6?"

A: "I think I need to talk with my wife about our diet and we would need to stop eating out so much."

Scaling confidence gives us important information about what we feel we *can* do (strengths, resources, abilities, and so on). It also helps break down what the next steps might look like and how we might go about those steps to increase the chance of success. One of the challenging thought traps we can get caught in is thinking about change as an either/or proposition. Either I follow the diet 100 percent and do it just right, or I don't. We think in dichotomous or black-and-white terms. As we consider change, it is important to scale our steps so that we can take a measured and tolerable risk while preserving our sense of confidence and stability. Thinking again about the stages of change discussed earlier, it is also important to plan for slips, relapses, and detours along the way. The mind-set has to be one of "I will try this step that I feel confident in taking, and I will learn about myself and what works or not as I do this."

To put this "change process" to work in your own life, first identify your core values and beliefs and compare and contrast this with your current situation and behavior. Next, determine the "why" of change or how important change is to you in a particular area. Finally, once you've identified your values and established a level of importance, now consider how confident you feel in making a step toward your desired goal and adjust that step until it feels within reach. With each attempt to move forward, consider the stages of change and look to learn from each effort to help you prepare for the next attempt. Continue this process with your values and goals in mind, and change will come. Here are some concrete steps, exercises, and resources to assist you in your efforts.

 ## ACTION ITEMS

Identify Stage of Change

Write the behavior you want to change here:

_____

Consider this behavior and draw a circle around the statement in the statement column below that best describes your stage of change:

Statement	Stage of Change	Question
"I would really like to but . . ."	Contemplation	"If I could overcome that barrier, what would I have to gain?"
"I have started taking steps."	Preparation	"What would be the next small step in the direction of my goal?"
"I've been doing it for the last three months or so."	Action	"How do I make sure to stick with it?"
"I've been doing it for at least six months."	Maintenance	"What benefits have I noticed so far?"
"I fell off the wagon."	Relapse	"What did I learn this time around?"

This will help you determine which stage of change you are at currently, and you can ask yourself the question in the "Question" column to determine what you need to do next to give yourself the motivation you need to proceed.

Let's consider an example that could be common to many of us: exercise.

Step 1: Identify the behavior you want to change: Increasing physical activity

"I would really like to, but I don't have time" (contemplation). If I could overcome that barrier, what would I have to gain? I'd probably have more energy and be more efficient."

Step 2: Value Sorting Exercise

Choose ten to fifteen values that are significant to you, and sort them in order of importance. Ask yourself how your current behavior is aligned or in conflict with your most important values. Ask yourself how your desired change or behavior is aligned or in conflict with your most important values. (Values: health, energy, efficiency. Current behavior: sedentary life.) For more information about value sorting, visit WholeFitWellness.com/special-appendices.html.

Step 3: Scale Importance and Confidence

As discussed earlier in the chapter, scaling questions can help to clarify readiness to change. Use the following scaling questions to identify your readiness.

- Example: Scaling Importance

    1. "On a scale from zero to ten (where zero is not important at all and ten is the most important thing), how important is it for you to _____?"

    2. "What makes it that number?"

    3. "Why not a lower number?"

    Q: "On a scale from zero to ten (where zero is not important at all and ten is the most important thing), how important is it for you to increase your physical activity?"

    A: "It is about a six."

    Q: "What makes it that number?"

    A: "I value health and fitness but I have been too busy at work to take care of myself."

    Q: "Why not a lower number?"

    A: "Because I remember how good I felt when I was working out consistently, and I know I am not getting any younger."

- Example: Scaling Confidence

    1. "On a scale from zero to ten (where zero is not confident at all and ten is the most confident), how confident do you feel about being able to _____?"

    2. "What makes it that number?"

    3. "Why not a lower number?"

    Q: "On a scale from zero to ten (where zero is not confident at all and ten is the most confident), how confident do you feel about being able to increase your physical activity?"

    A: "About a six."

    Q: "What makes it a six?"

    A: "If I set myself that goal, I would figure it out. I am really busy with work right now, so that makes it hard."

    Q: "Why not a four or a five?"

    A: "Because I have done it before, and it felt really good, so I could do it again."

Step 4: Taking Action!: DARN-CT

This next exercise will help give voice to your own change talk. The mnemonic DARN-CT (Desire, Ability, Reasons, Need, Commitment, Taking steps) is designed to help identify and evoke the various components of change talk. The research on change has shown that the more we talk about change and our reasons and desires to make a difference in our lives, the more likely we are to actually change.

Answer each of the following questions:

> "WE BECOME MORE COMMITTED TO THAT WHICH WE VOICE."[6]

1. Desire: *Why would I want to make this change?*

2. Ability: *How could I do it in order to succeed?*

3. Reason: *What are two or three good reasons to do it?*

4. Need: *What makes this change important to me?*

5. Commitment: *What do I intend to do?*

6. Taking steps: *What have I already tried or what am I willing to try?*

- Example
  - Desire
    Q: Why would I want to increase my physical activity?
    A: "I am tired of feeling tired, I want to feel fit."
  - Ability
    Q: How could I do it, in order to succeed?
    A: "I need to start slow, so I don't overdo it."
  - Reason
    Q: What are three good reasons to do increase my physical activity?
    A: "Increase health, fitness, and energy. And it could help my mood."
  - Need
    Q: What makes this change important to you?
    A: "I am getting older and my body is changing. I want to take better care of myself."
  - Commitment
    Q: What do you intend to do?
    A: "I am going to start walking every day."
  - Taking steps
    Q: What have you already tried or are willing to try?
    A: "I will park the farthest away from the entrance of the office building."

> "ONE DAY YOU FINALLY KNEW WHAT YOU HAD TO DO, AND BEGAN"[7]
>
> —MARY OLIVER

Once you've reflected on personal values and behavior, scaled importance, scaled confidence, and identified stages of change with a determination to begin, you are ready to set your goal. A final tool that can be helpful as you set your goal for change is to use another mnemonic called a SMART goal.[8] SMART goals are specific, measurable, attainable, realistic, and time-based. Once you have expressed a commitment and desire to change, you can set a SMART goal to guide the process.

- Example: Target behavior = increasing physical activity
  - **S (Specific):** I will start walking more during my work days
  - **M (Measurable):** I will use a phone app to count my steps and increase my average daily steps by one thousand steps this week.
  - **A (Attainable):** I will start parking farther away from the entrance of the office building, and I will take the stairs instead of the elevator.
  - **R (Realistic):** I will do it every work day unless it is raining.
  - **T (Time-based):** I will plot my steps every week for one month.

Notice that in the SMART goal example, the behavior change is paired with an existing behavior or routine. We also know from research on change that if we pair a new behavior with an existing one that is happening consistently (brushing teeth, parking in a lot for work, walking a dog after work, getting the mail, taking medication, and so on), we are more likely to be successful.

CONCLUSION

As a family therapist and family physician, we recognize there are cases when a person's best intentions, efforts, and motivation will not lead to change happening in ways that are satisfying to the individual or to those around them. In such cases, professional care and support may be necessary. Some changes are realized only through intensive psychotherapeutic treatment or medical attention and care. That said, we believe in the power of the human spirit and that the capacity for change lies within our physical (biological), mental (psychological), relational (sociological), and spiritual capacities and can be realized as we reach both within and toward those in our lives who love and care for us. We hope that the recommendations in this chapter will help guide your journey and process of change in ways that will be satisfying to you and others.

NOTES

1. John P. Kotter, *Leading Change* (Boston, MA: Harvard Business Review Press, 2012).

2. Stephen Covey, as quoted on Goodreads.com, accessed October 10, 2015, https://www.goodreads.com/quotes/126096-motivation-is-a-fire-from-within-if-someone-else-tries.

3. Heraclitus, as quoted on Goodreads.com, accessed October 10, 2015, https://www.goodreads.com/quotes/336994.

4. J. Prochaska, C. DiClemente, and J. Norcross, "In search of how people change: Applications to addictive behaviors," *American Psychologist* 47, no. 9 (1982) 1102–114.

5. S. Rollnick, W. Miller, and C. Butler, *Motivational Interviewing in Health Care: Helping patients change behavior* (New York: Guilford Press, 2008).

6. Julie Childers, Alda Maria Gonzaga, and Carla Spagnoletti, "Motivating the Motivational Interview: Teaching Residents to Empower Patients for Health Behavior Change," University of Pittsburgh, accessed October 10, 2015, connect.im.org/d/do/4142.

7. Mary Oliver, "The Journey," accessed October 10, 2015, http://www.poetryconnection.net/poets/Mary_Oliver/3124.

8. George T. Doran, "There's a S.M.A.R.T. Way to Write Management's Goals and Objectives," *Management Review*, 1981.

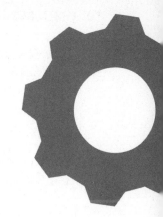

5 DISCOVERING OUR LIFE PURPOSE

BY W. JARED DUPREE, PHD, MBA

"SINCERITY AND TRUTH ARE THE BASIS OF EVERY VIRTUE."
—ATTRIBUTED TO CONFUCIUS

John (name and elements changed to protect confidentiality) was in his sixties and was sent to the weight loss program at Mercy Hospital in Manhattan, Kansas, because of the impact type 2 diabetes was having on his life. During our first meeting, it became obvious that he did not want to be there. His wife and primary care physician had "forced" him to come. I think he was expecting me to tell him to eat healthier, exercise more, and so on. He was pleasantly surprised that we ended up talking about his love for horses. He loved riding, raising horses, and being in a "ranch environment." I asked him when he had last spent time with his horses. "It's been months," he lamented, "and even then I really didn't enjoy myself that much."

"Why not?," I asked.

"I was thinking too much about work like I always do," he said. "It always gets in the way."

John was the owner and founder of a successful company, and that meant his lifestyle came with a lot of stress. I thought maybe he didn't have enough money to retire and enjoy his horses.

"No! I've got plenty of money," he said. If money was not the issue, then what was the problem?

I knew John needed to eat better, exercise, and lose weight, but I also knew me telling him to do what a dozen others had already counseled, nagged, and encouraged him to do would only add to his frustration.

"I have an idea, John. Rather than focusing on what you were 'forced' to come here for, why don't we do something different?" He was intrigued.

"Let's make the following goal for your program: increase your frequency and level of enjoyment with your horses," I suggested. He was floored! One, he liked the idea that I wouldn't be another person in his life hounding him and telling him what to do. And two, he really did want to be with his horses more often and enjoy them more when he was there. He was slightly confused though.

"I thought I was coming here to lose weight—what do my horses have to do with that?" he questioned.

I convinced him to trust me with the idea, "If within six weeks you don't feel like this program is worth it, then worst-case scenario is you got to spend some more time with your horses. I think in the end you may be surprised though. Deal?" He agreed.

Over the next six weeks, I discovered that he did not want to leave his position because he didn't feel anyone could replace him and then the business would go under and leave a lot of people unemployed. I also learned that he skipped meals during business hours and then ate a lot at night or sustained himself during the day with Coke or high-sugar foods. He ended up feeling extremely tired after these sugar rushes and would have low energy along with low motivation because he saw no way out of his current work dilemma. I also learned that when he was out at his ranch and riding, he typically enjoyed life more, ate better, and enjoyed working on the ranch (which meant he was burning calories). We helped him develop a leadership development program in his company. He was able to identify a young man that he felt had a lot of leadership potential as well as train others to take on leadership roles. As he delegated and trained more, he spent more time at his ranch with less worry. He ate better (something he already knew how to do), he exercised more (doing what he loved to do at his ranch), and he was able to enjoy himself (knowing there was a light at the end of the tunnel with his work situation). Guess what? He lost weight. Guess what else? We hardly ever talked about weight or eating or exercise. In the end, we aligned his own internal talents, passions, and goals with his life, and his body responded positively. In the end, we aligned his lifestyle with a life purpose that not only included spending time with his horses but also spending more time with his wife, kids, and grandkids. Helping him find his life purpose made all the difference.

Glenda (name and elements changed to protect confidentiality) was a university administrator who needed to lose weight and was prediabetic based on her eating habits and lack of exercise. Unlike John, she wanted to lose weight and came into the program voluntarily. However, as I got to know Glenda, it became clear that losing weight was really something her husband and others wanted more than she did. She did feel self-conscious about how she looked compared to years past. She did feel that when she was healthier she felt better. However, the stress of the job and her relationship with her husband was taking a toll. I asked about her kids and discovered she also had some grandkids. At that point, she really lit up! In only seconds, she went from a shamed woman giving a confession of her own faults to a proud grandmother, excited to tell me about her wonderful grandkids.

"My grandkids are my life!" she said. "They bring me more joy than anything I have right now."

I had another idea. "Glenda, our goal for your program is to increase the frequency and enjoyment of the time you spend with your grandkids. What do you think?" Similar to John, we went through the same type of questions as John on "How will that help me lose weight?" and "I'm paying a lot of money for this program; I don't want to waste my time." Similar to John, I convinced her to give me a try, and the worst that could happen is that she would spend some more time with her grandkids. Deal made.

As I worked with Glenda, I discovered that she really enjoyed getting on the floor with her grandkids to play with them. However, her weight and low energy made it difficult for her to fully experience her grandkids. She wished she had the energy and health to really spend some quality playtime with them. We needed to increase her energy level and help her body reach a level that could help her play. She also used soda and caffeine quite a bit to keep up her energy during the day but would experience a drop-off in energy at night or on the weekends. Some weekends she wouldn't get out of bed at all because she felt so tired.

Based on her own analysis of the situation, she decided to cut down on the Diet Cokes and eventually eliminate them all together. She also recognized she felt better after getting enough sleep and engaging in light activity. Obviously the caffeine started to impact her sleep on some level, but she also made some changes in her nighttime routine that helped her de-stress. She spent some time reading a favorite book, she took a hot bath, or she engaged in a hobby she enjoyed. This allowed her to let go of the worries of the day that seemed to stress her out and lead into a stressful night. She admitted she hated to exercise but knew that engaging in light activity helped her joints and energy levels. Knowing she loved to read, I suggested listening to a book on tape as she walked, with the goal that she could only listen to it as she walked. Based on the section of the book or excitement of the story, there were days she walked way beyond her typical thirty minutes so she could hear the rest of the story! Needless to say, her energy level went up, she slept better, her joints improved, her mood improved, and she was able to play with her grandkids more! By the way, she also lost weight.

During my time at Mercy Hospital, I worked with quite a few patients, and every single one lost a significant amount of weight. Yet, for most patients, the main goal that we wrote down didn't even use the phrase "lose weight." We helped them ride horses more and play on the floor with their grandkids.

What I have discovered as I have worked with patients and clients is that as we align ourselves with our discovered life purposes, other areas in our life seem to naturally fall into place. Our bodies respond better, we develop healthier habits, our minds are clearer, we our more motivated and happy, and our relationships improve. It is almost like our body, mind, and soul were waiting for us to do what we always knew we should be doing. Our body, mind, and soul respond quickly like we have done this before, and we are just getting back into it. Maybe we *are* returning to something we forgot or "lost" along the way.

My hope for this chapter, and ultimately for this book is to give you some ideas and methods you can use to discover life's purpose and then align your lifestyle choices with that purpose. In other words, I want to help you identify how your talents, strengths, passions, values, and beliefs matter, and how to best employ them in your current stage of life to bring yourself joy and fulfilment. I want to help you find more happiness, which, in the end, will lead to better health and wellness. Many of the concepts addressed by Mike and Catalina in the previous chapter can be translated into discovering and being able to articulate a life purpose. Understanding what motivates us to change often unlocks elements of that purpose.

DISCOVERING YOUR LIFE PURPOSE

From a philosophical standpoint, discovering your life purpose is sometimes described as discovering your "true self" and living it. Some describe the process as living a sincere life. The word *sincere* has some interesting origin stories. It is unclear if they are actually true, but I think the message provides a great illustration. The story goes that ancient sculptors would use wax to cover up the flaws of stone statues, and that wax would end up melting in the sun after being sold. Thus, buyers would request sculptures "sin cera," which means "without wax." Whether or not the story is true, I like the imagery. Sincerity from that standpoint would suggest a person that is presenting their true self— not a misrepresentation or facade of self. What does that really mean?

For one thing, I think the discovery process is not a one-time event but rather a process of rediscovery over and over again through a person's life. What does that discovery process look like? For me, it is a reflection on what is important in life as I consider where I am in my journey, where I have been, and where I am going. It is common to forget the big picture. An inspired leader in his old age once told me, "I am the happiest man on earth because I see the big picture." More recently, my wife's grandmother in her nineties taught me a great lesson. She mentioned her desire to downsize and simplify because she wouldn't be taking much with her to the other side. I have always heard that notion expressed, both in religious contexts and in day-to-day conversations, that "you can't take it with you," but I really didn't think about it seriously until she helped me understand the concept literally. None of us will take anything with us after this life except our intelligence, memories, and relationships. The question comes to mind then, "Why work so hard to build and obtain things that don't matter much?" We all obviously need to make a living, take care of the necessities of life, make the bed, clean the car, and so on. But how do we spend our time? What is time best used for? What are we trying to build? As I have worked with many people on some of those same questions, I have discovered most people are trying to make sense of some core needs and wants. I have made my own list throughout the years of the most common core "true needs"; these tend to be the opposite of the most common core pains people are trying to avoid:

I feel rejected.	I want to feel accepted.
I feel unneeded.	I want to feel needed.
I feel unimportant.	I want to feel important.
I feel unwanted.	I want to feel wanted.
I feel guilty.	I want to feel forgiveness.
I feel lonely.	I want to feel connection.
I feel disrespected.	I want to feel respected.

So one of the first steps in discovering your life purpose may be to think of the big picture and what is important to you. Some of the core pains can give light to some common themes that people discover:

1. The feeling of being needed or important often translates to a desire to offer talents, strengths, and passions to others. It can also mean offering service or helping others.

2. The feeling of being wanted or feeling connected or even feeling forgiveness generally is based on the quality of one's relationships.

3. The feelings of acceptance and respect can reflect a desire to share and develop thoughts, talents, opinions, feelings, and experiences with integrity and honesty, and without fear.

Thus, I have discovered that most people discover that their life purposes have to do with one of three areas:

1. Sharing their time, talents, and strengths with others in order to help them and our world

2. Developing lasting relationships with family and friends or even a higher power that rely on both connection and healing as they work through the challenges of life

3. Improving themselves as they continue to learn and grow and share that growth with others

In very simple terms, you will likely be drawn to one, two, or all three of the following areas: (1) personal growth, (2) service, and (3) relationships.

PERSONAL GROWTH

It is common for people to try to achieve personal gain for external reasons. For example, consider the student that goes to medical school because her parents want her to (external desire of someone else), or the employee that works at a particular job that he hates because he needs to pay the bills (external reward). It is not necessarily wrong to seek personal gain for external reasons. However, researchers have found that those who engage in activities for internal reasons are more likely to be productive, enjoy what they do, and actually achieve their personal or financial goals sooner. Thus, one way to increase personal growth is to discover one's internal motivations, passions, talents, and strengths.

Mihaly Csikszentmihalyi is a Hungarian psychologist that studied at the University of Chicago and is considered one of the fathers of positive psychology (the scientific study of understanding and achieving life satisfaction). He developed the concept of *flow*. He provides some additional insight into how aspects of motivation can help us discover our personal passions. When someone experiences flow, they are fully immersed in an activity, feeling energized and completely involved in what they are doing.

Some of the common characteristics of flow across groups include

- sense of timelessness, or time passing rapidly
- loss of reflective consciousness, or living in the moment
- intense focus
- sense of person control and freedom
- intrinsic motivation or autotelic experience

Some people describe it as "being in the zone." It's like when Michael Jordan would get into the "zone," hitting every shot and seeming unstoppable.

Or a composer may experience flow as ideas *flow* quickly and easily as masterpieces are created. Even a mother can experience flow as she connects with her child and experiences a moment of timelessness and intense joy. In fact, Csikszentmihalyi studied various groups like biker gangs, monks, athletes, and artists and found that each of these groups experienced flow at times. Even more profoundly, he discovered that the experience of flow is controllable. In other words, there are things each of us can do to increase our chances of entering into flow more often. When helping others consider their areas of flow, I tend to ask common questions:

1. What are you most passionate about or gets you excited the most?

2. When do you enjoy yourself the most?

3. When you were younger, what did you dream about or what were your passions? Do those dreams tap into interests or passions you haven't had a chance to engage in or explore?

4. Are there times you get in the zone? Are there times you feel closer to your true self?

As you consider the answers to these questions, you may be able to pinpoint your opportunities for flow. Some people identify a hobby or interest, while others identify an activity or even a relationship. If you can successfully identify times when you most consistently experience "flow," you will have discovered important clues that will lead you to clarifying your life purpose. Researchers have noted that when people align their passions, talents, and strengths and make those part of their everyday activities through their work, relationships, roles, and hobbies, they experience more intensive, directed personal growth. In fact, it is likely you will begin to excel in areas that others will notice seem to be a perfect fit or easy choice. If one of your life purposes is achieving personal growth, identifying activities where you feel "flow" may be the key to unlocking a future path that will bring you fulfilment and a sense of purpose.

GIVING SERVICE

A common life purpose for many includes giving service to others. A wealthy gentleman gave me the key to purposeful service when he said, "Everyone wishes they could get to a point where they could give vast amounts of money to the needy and help others. But what most people don't know is that we can all give service, even if we aren't wealthy, and sometimes that type of service is more valuable than money." This is a profound observation. We don't need to be wealthy to have a significant impact for good in the world. If your life purpose is to give tremendous service, you do not necessarily need to develop great wealth first. I have often made the mistake of looking toward the future too much and saying to myself, "When I am older and more well-off, then I will have time for _____ or be able to help with _____." Lately, I have realized I enjoy serving others, and there are small and simple things we can do each day as we interact with one another that can help others immensely.

Many of us miss opportunities to serve and connect because we are too preoccupied about the future or the past. We miss the moment. We can learn from the past and always plan for the future, but living in the *now* can help us make a difference. Flow through service occurs through the service itself. The enjoyment is found in the activity.

RELATIONSHIPS

I have had the chance to work with a number of people who are on their "deathbed" as they reminisce about their lives, and our conversations often turn to relationships. It is not uncommon for people to think about a spouse, child, friend or other important relationships. When people have someone from whom they can seek comfort, safety, and loyalty, they are happier. When we have people in our lives with whom we can share who we are, seek to understand them, and seek to be understood, we feel more accepted and connected. We find solace and joy in the fact that we are loved for who we are and that we are unique *and* similar to others. It is through our connections that we invite understanding and peace. Thus, for some of us we may find that our life purpose is building bridges between others and finding connections to strengthen our humanity.

There will be some of us who choose to be nurturers or healers. Many of the authors writing this book fall into this category. They feel a need to reach out to others and help heal their souls and help them build their own connections. Interestingly, I have discovered that when I wade too long in the waters of healing others, I will become drained. I have learned the importance of trying to build and maintain appropriate boundaries so that I can heal others when I need to but also take a "time-out" to rest and be healed myself.

Finally, many of us will find purpose in connecting with a higher power. We will discuss in more detail the importance of spirituality in our lives in chapter 14. It is important to note that one of the reasons many of us choose relationships as part of our life purpose is that it can provide us with a means to heal and find meaning in life. A relationship with a higher power like a Heavenly Father, Savior, Holy Spirit, God, or even nature can also provide us with the opportunity to heal and find meaning. This healing power of relationships will be discussed more in chapter 12. In general, we are able to access a power greater than ourselves and seek understanding and value through our relationship with a higher power.

Most of us will find that our life purpose will fall into all three areas: (1) personal growth, (2) service, and (3) relationships. Many discover that their life purpose is founded in all three areas but in specific ways that make sense only to them. For example, I am personally motivated by growth in terms of wanting to learn and discover what "makes us tick." I research and write about creativity, life enjoyment, and innovation because I enjoy learning about what helps us surpass our own expectations. But I am also motivated by service and enjoy helping others discover their own passions and use their innovative abilities to teach or develop products and services that help people. Finally, I am also motivated by relationships—not only with my immediate and extended family but also with my ancestors. I have an intense love for family history, and as I discover the legacies of my ancestors, I feel a deep connection to them. I am equally motivated by continually developing and refining my relationship with my Heavenly Father. I am just beginning to understand my relationship with a higher power.

It is important at this point, to remind readers of the concept of flow and intrinsic motivation. Remember, when we are able to identify those areas in our life that seemed to give us greater enjoyment out of an internal love or desire to engage in that activity, it is likely we are edging up on our life purpose. These type of internal motivations go beyond our physical needs (food, water, or sex) or our senses (taste, touch, and so on). They even go beyond our immediate emotional reactions. Rather, they tend to live deeper inside of us in a place that is more lasting, meaningful, and sincere. Thus, a relational connection is more than the immediate pleasure of sexual intimacy, service is more than accepting an assignment to help someone out, and personal growth is more than learning a new skill. Those parts of life are usually appendages to our deeper life purpose. I'm all for helping others, good sex, and learning new skills! However, your life purpose will likely be more. Personal growth will be about finding your true self and sharing that with the world even in the face of opposition. Service will be about gaining a deep love for others. Relational connection will be about sharing the good, the bad, and the ugly with those special people in your life.

 ## ACTION ITEMS

I invite you to consider your life purposes. It is likely you will have more the one; it is likely that this may change or evolve over time. Thus, your homework for this chapter is simple!

1. **Journal or write down your life purpose.** As we discussed, consider the main needs and wants you have in life. Consider the areas of your life that bring you more peace or life enjoyment. Consider how those areas relate to personal growth, service, or connecting with others. Try to write down your thoughts about your life purpose in either a journal or a place that you could review often. Consider reviewing and adjusting over time.

2. **Share that life purpose with the special people in your life.** Consider sharing this life purpose with others like a spouse, partner, friend, or even higher power. See what they think, and seek out suggestions about how they feel your life purpose aligns with how they see you. You may be surprised with what they have to say.

CONCLUSION

In conclusion, your life purpose in many ways will be the key in providing life balance and enjoyment to your life. It will help you make decisions, prioritize, and learn to say yes or no, depending on the situation. As discussed, some of us have a difficult time saying yes to things because we think we might fail, believe we don't have the time, or feel it is not important. Others of us have a difficult time saying no to people who request our time or to activities in our life because we feel obligated somehow. Knowing your life purpose will help you know when to say yes because it fits who you are, which will lead to more success and enjoyment in that area. Knowing your life purpose will help you know when to say no to those areas that take up time and energy for things that don't matter.

Finding life purpose can also help us align how we spend our time and what becomes important to us. We will learn in later chapters about the importance of eating well, engaging in physical activity, and treating our bodies well. When we have a life purpose, the nutrition, fitness, and other health-related activities become areas that help support our life purpose. It is important that we connect our behaviors and choices to the bigger picture. Everything is connected. How we eat, spend our time, and engage in activities can all be tied to our life purpose. Those behaviors will either support your life purpose or derail you from your true path, but finding that path is exciting and purposeful. In fact, it makes *all* the difference.

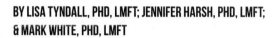

6 MINDFULNESS

TAKING BACK YOUR LIFE

BY LISA TYNDALL, PHD, LMFT; JENNIFER HARSH, PHD, LMFT;
& MARK WHITE, PHD, LMFT

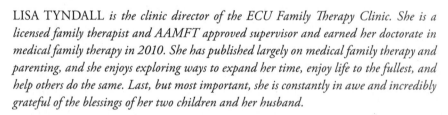

"I WOULD LOVE TO LIVE LIKE A RIVER FLOWS, CARRIED BY
THE SURPRISE OF ITS OWN UNFOLDING."[1]
—JOHN O'DONOHUE

LISA TYNDALL *is the clinic director of the ECU Family Therapy Clinic. She is a licensed family therapist and AAMFT approved supervisor and earned her doctorate in medical family therapy in 2010. She has published largely on medical family therapy and parenting, and she enjoys exploring ways to expand her time, enjoy life to the fullest, and help others do the same. Last, but most important, she is constantly in awe and incredibly grateful of the blessings of her two children and her husband.*

JENNIFER HARSH *earned her PhD from East Carolina University in medical family therapy. She directs the behavioral medicine program for the division of general internal medicine at the University of Nebraska Medical Center. Professionally, she is interested in assisting families in coping with illness experiences and in creating useful strategies for integrating behavioral medicine into primary care settings. Jennifer enjoys spending time with family and friends and participating in activities that allow her to spend time on a lake, river, or ocean.*

MARK WHITE *obtained a PhD from Kansas State University in human ecology, with a specialization in marriage and family therapy. His research has examined how individuals manage life with a chronic illness. One of his professional emphases has been helping individuals find meaning and make sense of the challenges facing them. He directs the marriage and family therapy doctoral program at Northcentral University and is the manager of the Vernal Center for Couples and Families. Mark lives in the Uintah Basin and enjoys hiking, cooking, being a grandfather, reading, and spending time with his family.*

Editor's note: These authors have worked for years with people who experience chronic illness, brain injuries, or other difficult medical conditions. They have discovered ways to help their clients cope and receive support. We are grateful for the rich experience and insight they bring to this important topic of mindfulness.

INTRODUCTION

Have you ever been at one of your child's sporting events, thinking about all you have to accomplish before bedtime? Have you ever been eating lunch with a friend, and been not wholly invested in the conversation because you were worrying about the big work project due the next day? Have you ever found yourself driving through a scenic area only to realize later that you have almost no recollection of what you passed along the way?

If these scenarios sound familiar, you're not alone. Thinking about the next thing we have to do or the past thing we regret is common. More "seasoned" people try to warn us: "It goes so fast! Your children will be grown before you know it!" With a gulp, a sense of panic and fear washes over me, and for a second I hold my breath as I realize how quickly life passes. There is a looming fear of losing time with my children, not developing my talents enough, not having time to develop any hobbies. I worry about getting to the end of my life not having paid enough attention to living my life well. The answer to this painful dilemma is to learn to use the tool of *mindfulness*. While we cannot slow time down, we can discernibly expand the time by paying closer attention to what is going on *in the moment*.

Mindfulness is a misunderstood concept in our culture, often linked to "weirdos" who eat granola and practice yoga daily or who wear long robes and walk around chanting. If you're convinced that becoming *mindful* isn't really for you, keep reading while we convince you otherwise.

Simply stated, mindfulness is paying attention, on purpose, to what one is experiencing *right now*—in this moment.[2] Essentially, the idea of mindfulness is to bring awareness back to your own everyday experiences,[3] but this awareness is more than a thought process, it is a *being* process. Can you picture a lamp with a flexible light pole? The light typically is shining out, focused on the external surroundings. Thanks to this light, you are fully aware of what is in front of you and to the side of you and behind you, but your awareness of what is happening inside of you is dim. Now, imagine bending that light pole around and shining that light, back onto the person who turned it on, shining that light on you and your experience—not just your thoughts but also your experience of that moment. This *bending back the light*[4] symbolizes shining the light on the present moment so that it can be fully appreciated and embraced.

Mindfulness has become a hot topic for those who study wellness.[5] Note that academic publications on mindfulness have gone from an annual publication rate of zero in 1980 to 350 by 2010. Mindfulness advocates continue to add to the body of research that asserts that developing mindfulness can help improve quality of life, quality of parenting,[6] eating,[7] chronic pain,[8, 9] and stress levels.[10, 11] Regardless of the topic area, the practice of mindfulness is moving full steam ahead in American culture.

Mindfulness had its roots in Buddhism twenty-five centuries ago, and as different branches of Buddhism have developed over the centuries, mindfulness has remained a core teaching.[12] Its increasing popularity soon spread outside of religious boundaries,[13] and it is now practiced by many outside of a specific religion or ideological background[14] because proponents the world over have recognized the benefits of mindfulness practice for relieving suffering and increasing well-being.

So how does mindfulness relieve suffering? While *suffering* may seem like a strong word, consider the idea that missing out on an interaction with a loved one due to anxiety about an event the next day or a project for work is a form of suffering. Being emotionally or mentally transported (distracted by worry or concern) and missing out on the moment you have *now* because you are worried about a moment that has passed or has yet to come is a form of loss. Hurting and isolating yourself from friends and loved ones because of an illness, mental or physical, is a form of suffering. With depression as one of the most common mental disorders in America,[15] and with ads for medications for depression and anxiety filling our television screens, it is easy to see that most people can relate to some level of difficulty or suffering in an area in their life.

In our world of selfies, status updates, and perpetual pings and whistles alerting us to the next event or activity on the calendar, we have largely lost the art of truly being *in* each moment of our lives. It is this "being" that, at the end of it all, we do not want to miss. Even the phrase human *being* should give us pause to remember that it is this *being* that is most important. We are not human doings. So in order to help you understand mindfulness, it might be helpful to start with an illustration:

Marissa has been worried about an upcoming biology test and decides a nice, green salad will help her feel better, so she stops to take time to make one for herself. An hour later, she closes her biology textbook, still thinking about that salad when she realizes that she actually already ate it. The empty plate is at the corner of her desk, along with a bag of chocolate truffles (her favorite) that she had wolfed down distractedly as she was studying, never taking time to actually savor either one of them.

In this case, the salad and the chocolate truffles represent the *It*. In an attempt to not miss the *It* (the crunch of the spiced croutons and the flavor of the dressing on her salad or the chocolatey smoothness of the truffles), mindfulness practice would have enabled Marissa to stop briefly, focus on what she was eating, enjoy the moment, and then return to her studying, refreshed and ready to concentrate. Mindfulness practice, either formal or informal, can be a great help. It is an opportunity to simply *be*, without *doing*. Kabat-Zinn refers to this as "non-doing" or "practicing being,"[16] and while that may sound simple, it can be quite difficult in our constantly moving culture. The benefits of slowing down and practicing mindfulness can be exponential. When we increase our being and are attuned to our experiences, we become more aware of our mind, body, relationships and, as a result, needs and overall well-being.[17] Even as individuals, we are part of a larger picture, and when we are more aware of our own being, we can more fully connect with those around us.

PRINCIPLES OF MINDFULNESS

Kabat-Zinn listed seven basic principles that seem to have made it into the contemporary concept and work of mindfulness: Nonjudgment, patience, beginners' mind, trust, nonstriving, acceptance, and letting go.[18] Other themes run through author and Zen monk, Thich Nhat Hanh's work, such as interdependence, impermanence, and living in the present.[19] Below you will find a brief introduction to just a few of the main principles of mindfulness (awareness, nonjudging, responding versus reacting, acceptance, nonstriving), and we encourage you to seek out the original texts listed at the end of this chapter and suggestions for further reading for additional information.

Awareness of the need for being mindful in daily life is a critical element to any mindfulness practice. It is likely that if you are reading this chapter, you already have some awareness that something is missing or that some change is needed in your life. Maybe you feel particularly rushed on a day-to-day basis. Maybe you have noticed an increase in the tension in your shoulders that possibly results in headaches. Maybe you have recognized an increase in conflictual interactions with loved ones. These are common experiences for many. Unpleasant events and interactions happen to everyone.[20]

What causes suffering (and this is one element that mindfulness can help us with) is the way we *think* about that suffering. We don't always have control over *what* is happening, but we do have control over the way we choose to *experience* what is happening. We can work to become aware that it is not what is happening that makes us feel emotion or physical pain. Rather, our perceptions, thoughts, and our awareness about them are what produce these sensations. Even Shakespeare recognized this power when he said in Hamlet, "For there is nothing either good or bad, but thinking makes it so."[21]

This judging about events, thoughts, and actions has a powerful impact, and mindfulness can help us slow down and choose how we'd like to respond. Kabat–Zinn identified nonjudging as one of the most important tenets of mindfulness practice.[22] Nonjudging can be accomplished by paying attention to internal judgments and reactions, and learning to take a step back and observe them instead of reacting to them. Becoming less preoccupied with placing judgments on ongoing experiences can allow an individual to find calm and acceptance.[23] One of the best places to start is simply paying attention to how quickly our mind can move, even with relation to something as simple as a food choice.

Here's another example: Consider John, who is working to lose weight. He came home from work hungry, and the first thing he encountered in the pantry was a bag of Oreos. Faced with that indulgent food choice, he decided that he was so famished, he'd go ahead and eat a handful. The judgment or value John places on that food choice can have a powerful impact on his experience. He can choose to label or judge himself as "bad" for failing to control his impulse to gobble down cookies, which could lead to his giving up on his attempt to become healthier as a whole because he then labels himself as weak or overindulgent. That judgment can be so powerful that it even becomes about John himself, not just about his food choice.

As another option, John can see the food as simply food, and eating cookies as an experience and let himself enjoy the experience without judgment. Chances are that if the latter is chosen, he can move on to the next experience, without carrying any judgment with him, and continue with his healthy eating at the next meal. If a judgment is attributed to that experience, then the Oreos are long gone, but the suffering attached to the negative judgment lingers and taints future events. So one step to ending the suffering is ending the judgment.

Slowing down and becoming aware of our thoughts and the judgments associated with those thoughts allows us the ability to respond versus react. Using mindfulness in daily life can help people focus on experienced thoughts and feelings moment to moment, allowing for the ability to take a moment, and respond to outside stimuli instead of immediately reacting. The clarity that comes from witnessing our experiences allows for more control in making positive choices and changes in life.[24] It allows us to function as our best selves, extending a sense of loving-kindness, when we can sit back and extend compassion to others because judging our experiences is not getting in the way.[25]

Increased awareness, nonjudgment, and having the ability to respond out of our best selves combined with an acceptance of what the situation actually is allows us to embrace our present moment. Remember, the importance of embracing that present moment—of being mindful of that moment—is that it allows us to not feel as if life is passing us by. It allows us the ability to almost expand our sense of time and experience. We also move toward an ability to accept and be compassionate with others through this process.

All too often, American culture is about the drive for success, which means different things to different people, but it rarely means accepting what currently exists. We seem to almost always find fault with our current situation. The drive to look good, make money, and have the perfect romantic relationship can lead to a great deal of stress and unhappiness in our lives. We may spend unnecessary time and brain space on looking for the job that will make us rich instead of the job that is meaningful to us. We may spend hours of screen time on social media sites, looking into the lives of others, as we attempt to emulate the aspects of our friends' lives that we deem desirable. Our lives are full of "shoulds" and "have tos," and we create goals that seem to be the key to happiness, assuming that once we will have accomplished those goals, then, and only then, we can finally accept and appreciate our lot in life. This sense of striving for the next best thing goes back centuries; in fact, the Buddhist word *tanha* refers to an unquenchable desire that leads to suffering.[26] In a practice of mindfulness, we are working toward a sense of nonstriving. We can find much more contentment and fullness in our present moment when we stop senseless striving and accept where we are in the here and now.

This drive distracts us from paying attention to what is going on in our lives—what is actually happening right now for us. Each moment we are in is the only moment we have to live. We will never be living in tomorrow, and we will never be living in "a year from now when I have a better job." What can complicate it further is the idea that we connect that lacking or that yearning for something that we think is missing, to our character or something that is unchangeable within us.[27] We can take one moment in time, connect it to who we are as a person, and then it gets dragged into future events that have yet to happen.

Take for example, a pain experienced by a runner or a casual athlete. On a recent morning run, I [LT] felt a sharp pain in my left knee. The pain was such that I could not really fully extend my knee, so almost immediately, I began to worry. I created a brain process that told me, "This sharp pain is going to lead to surgery, and I may never be able to run again." As if that was not enough momentary suffering, I placed a further judgment on that pain by thinking about the fact that I could lose the companionship of my friends who were also runners and that I'd never again win a medal or improve my

PR. Because of my drive to continue this practice of running and because of what it means to me to be a runner, I increased my suffering by imagining a scenario that I might somehow lose that status and that label. I fired the "second arrow of suffering" so quickly that the pain in my knee was magnified, and I lost any hope of enjoying what was left of that beautiful morning exercise.

What I could have chosen, had I had a greater sense of awareness of my thoughts (and had I given myself time to respond to my thoughts rather than immediately reacting), was an opportunity to acknowledge that I had a pain that morning. With that, I could have accepted that pain in that moment for what it was. It simply meant I might need to walk more slowly that morning. Then, I could have gone on with my day. I have run since then with no pain at all. Those judgments, that lack of acceptance of myself and my process, and that need to continue striving and achieving the goal of being "a runner" created my own suffering. It was a choice I made. And so with mindfulness we can make a different choice and see that there is no pressure to be a certain way or achieve a certain level of something. *There is no goal in mindfulness, because it is a process.* There is nothing we are striving for, and there is no place we are trying to be, we just need to simply learn the practice of being still, accepting where we are, and extending that loving-kindness to ourselves and others.

These changes that are made through the practice of mindfulness do not happen in a vacuum. We, as family therapists by trade, believe that each person is part of several systems of relationships, our family typically being the primary network. Teachers of mindfulness also see this sense of interconnectedness and see that as we become more aware of our own needs, we are better able to work to benefit those around us even more.[28] Contemporary researchers have demonstrated the benefits of mindfulness practice for couples and families.[29] Thus far, researchers have found that couples who practiced mindfulness reported increased relationship satisfaction, better response skills in stressful situations, and increased self-control, and they were better able to communicate with their partner effectively.[30] Another study found that couples practicing mindfulness were more able to cope with stress and had higher relationship satisfaction than couples that did not practice mindfulness.[31] Families may also benefit from mindfulness practices. Specifically, parents who practice mindfulness reported being better able to connect on a deeper level with their child.[32] It is these connections—this ability to be present—that we so often find missing in our lives. Mindfulness can be instrumental in closing that gap. In a meditation contained in the book *Your True Home,* we read, "Breathing with awareness, we generate our energy of mindfulness, and we can have insight into how to handle our suffering and that of the other person's suffering with compassion."[33] It seems that through a practice of mindfulness, we can work to alleviate our suffering and help others alleviate their own suffering as well, through the nurturing of our compassion for them and the nurturing of our relationships with them.

CASE EXAMPLES

To illustrate how mindfulness can be used, we wanted to provide you with a couple of case studies. The information and names have been changed to protect confidentiality.

Luke

Luke had just started his dream job. He had been looking forward to this position for years! He was even happy to move halfway across the country for this job. As he began his new position, he learned about all of his various tasks and responsibilities and discovered that there were a lot of people who were depending on him to make good decisions and to keep projects moving toward completion.

He found that during work, while at home, and even when waking up in the middle of the night, he couldn't find a way to release the pressure in his shoulders and found that he was unable to take deep breaths. From the time he woke up to the time he went to bed, he felt keyed up.

Also, he found that he couldn't stop mentally reviewing his to-do list repeatedly while outside of work. When he found himself thinking about work while having a serious conversation with his partner, he knew something had to change. He had heard about mindfulness meditation from a coworker a few years ago. At the time, he had no desire to meditate. It was a foreign concept to him, he thought it was a bit "hippie," and he didn't think he had a need. Now, he thought, Why not give it a shot? He searched for "mindfulness meditation" online and found a few examples. He began listening to a short five-minute meditation each morning before work and each night before bed.

He found that the more he tried to pay attention to each moment, the less he worried about what might happen the next day at work or whether he completed all of the tasks for the day. He also found he was more able to pay attention to his loved ones. When he was having conversations, he actually listened to what the other person was saying. He still has some tension in his body and still became short of breath. But he is more able to be present in his daily life and is less bothered by his tension and worries.

He plans to keep listening to these meditations and try to find ways to practice being present. When he drives, he pays attention to what is going on around him—the trees blowing and the cityscape in the distance. When he washes dishes, he pays attention to the water running over his hands, and the way the plates look while he cleans them. He notices the food he is eating, savoring each bite rather than mindlessly eating while reading or watching television. These activities help him to remember to pay attention to what is going on in each moment in his life.

Ann

Ann is the working mother of three school-aged children. Ann is middle-aged and has been married to the same man for twenty-two years. She would describe herself as ordinary, and her daily life as somewhat routine. However, Ann has struggled with the same twenty pounds her entire adult life. Not only does she battle the extra weight, but more recently she finds herself short on patience with herself and her family. It is all just too much for her to manage some days, and yet she feels guilty for saying that when she knows many people would love to have her mundane problems.

She reaches out for a therapy appointment, not even sure why because nothing is terribly wrong. She just has a nagging feeling of dread some days, and other days she just feels tense inside. She thinks perhaps medication might help—a referral to a psychiatrist for an anti-depressant or anti-anxiety, anti-something medicine will do the trick. After attending the first few sessions, Ann and her therapist begin to explore creating a practice of mindfulness. Ann is resistant at first because, let's face it, one more thing to have to remember to carve time out for is not on her list of favorites right now. But she trusts the therapist and so begins to participate in the out-of-session homework activities.

Her first assignment is to begin increasing her awareness of just how her body feels when she senses the tension. The therapist reminds her to try to notice what is going on when she feels tense. Over a period of weeks, Ann notices that she is tense when thinking about planning the week, the to-do list, or trying to get from point A to point B. She starts to notice an increasing physical tension in her shoulders and realizes that this could be related to those nagging headaches. Oddly enough, she also realizes that there are times she is holding her breath. What in the world could she be holding her breath for? It is almost as if the underlying tension generated by her worries about yesterday and tomorrow is being transmitted directly into her body, and she is holding her breath waiting for the next shoe to drop. In session, Ann begins to talk about her breathing and how that has become a concern for her, and the therapist suggests practicing taking deep breaths in the very same moment when she realizes that she is holding the breath. Not just gasps of air, but deep, slow, big belly breaths. Ann begins to tackle this when she feels that tension building in her shoulders, as she checks in with her breathing, and she feels a great release of tension as she takes that deep breath.

Over a period of weeks, Ann starts to notice that she is slowing down in certain scenarios when she used to become tense and short-tempered. She is starting to put the tension in its place and be more mindful of the way she wants to live, making conscious choices of her interactions with her loved ones. She even realizes that she had previously developed a mindless habit of snacking when she was tense, and she no longer finds herself standing in front of the pantry trying to sooth those worries, because the breath has filled that space. She chooses not to weigh herself—even after weeks of slowly developing a habit of being mindful about her eating—because she simply feels good about the choices she is making and she wants to practice that sense of loving-kindness to herself—the same loving-kindness she's able to extend to others more often. There are days when she struggles and still finds herself holding her breath, but those days, too, she can just notice that held breath and let it go, because the next moment is here and she is ready to embrace it.

ACTION ITEMS

We hope at this point this chapter has inspired or sparked an interest in mindfulness. We also know that making changes, even ones that we desperately want, can be an uphill battle. But we would like to encourage you to entertain making a few small changes, perhaps beginning one step at a time. Please keep in mind the principles above and that there is really no goal in the practice of mindfulness. It is a practice—a process, not a destination that you can check off your to-do list when you have achieved it. Remember to keep in mind to accept where you are in your practice, without judgment and with a heaping dose of loving-kindness toward yourself. If you can do so, your mindfulness efforts will grow and benefit you and those you love.

The action items below can be inserted into a formal or an informal practice of mindfulness. Mindfulness is often viewed as a repetitive practice, but this repetition can come in a variety of ways, including focusing on one thing at a time, repetitive thoughts or mantras, repetitive observance of the breath, or observance of thoughts without judgment.[34] It is this repetition and systematic practice[35] that is so important to retraining our ways of being. Allow yourself to return to developing your awareness and practice with ease and acceptance. Hanh references the beauty of simply being present with daily moments, for example while walking, washing dishes, sitting at a stoplight, and so on; you decide what is important to you and what will work for you.[36] You can pick the way you want to start, and there really is no end to the beauty this beginning will bring.

1. Attention

Paying attention and increasing awareness is a wonderful place to start your journey toward mindfulness. There is a range of ways you can begin to increase your awareness. Some people find it helpful to set aside a brief period of the day, often at the beginning their day, with even a small increment of five minutes, to sit with themselves and shine that light on their current experience. During this time, we encourage you to just watch the thoughts that come in and out of your consciousness and be aware them, aiming not to judge them, and not worrying about your "proficiency at mindfulness meditation." Just simply be. Kabat Zinn emphasizes the importance of this awareness in his book *Full Catastrophe Living,* when he writes, "Just being aware of the mind that thinks it knows all the time is a major step toward learning how to see through your opinions and perceive things as they actually are."[37]

Another option is to use a marker of some sort—a way to remind yourself during the day—to stop and pay attention to your current experience. One way to do this might be to wear a certain piece of jewelry that when you look at it, it reminds you to take stock and slow down in that moment to bend back that light. Others might chose to write and post a note on a place where you spend a lot of time, perhaps the bathroom mirror, the kitchen sink, or maybe even in the shower, as on-the-go reminders of taking time to be still in those moments and see where your thoughts lead you.

Last, another option is just to say to yourself now that you are going to try and remember throughout your day to pay more attention to your thoughts and your sense of being, to be more mindful in general. See, this is not goal-focused; this is just about what works for you and what you think will, eventually lead you on the path toward being able to *be* more than *do*. This action item should not be something to check off your list. Please use one of these examples or a combination of whatever works for you. There is no right or wrong. We are hoping to simply notice thoughts and feelings without placing judgment on them; that is the only intended "goal."[38]

2. Breath

Closely tied to the importance of bringing awareness to our thoughts is bringing awareness to our breath. Our breath and our being are so intimately connected that we bet you will find it hard not to connect action item one and two, but you can try. Our breath is powerful. It is what signals the beginning of life and the end of life and yet it is continually underestimated. Technically in Westernized language, our breath can assist us in switching from our sympathetic nervous system to our parasympathetic nervous system by helping regulate the levels of oxygen and carbon dioxide in our bodies. However, in our go-go-go world, with the constant stimulation, perceived and real threats, and distractions, we often stay in that sympathetic or stressed mode, deteriorating our minds, bodies, and families.

Similar to increasing your awareness and attention to your thoughts, you can simply choose a different point of entry and begin to pay attention to your breath. I [LT] have found great relief instantly in beginning to pay attention to my breath. A good deep belly breath can relax muscles and bring a tremendous sense of relief to an anxiety-filled moment. Breathing is a grounding experience that brings you back in touch with what your body is sensing and feeling, and yes, being! It brings your whole experience back into your body, when so often our mind is elsewhere, focused on the past or the future. So rarely are we existing mindfully in the only moment we truly have—the present.

A good deep breath is an important skill to master. As you inhale through your nose, it involves pushing out the belly in a way that allows the lungs to fully expand. When the "in" breath comes, the belly goes out, not the rib cage, and then flattens with a full exhale through the mouth. Similar to your attention to thoughts, we encourage you to take action with your breath in a way that works for you and that feels doable. You can set aside a set time to focus on the breath. Practitioners range in the length of time, but feel free to start with as brief a time as possible. Oddly enough, it can feel difficult to spend time just being. An informal practice throughout the day, with purposeful reminders or with a general attempt to pay more attention to the breath can all be ways to take action and incorporate this practice in a way that benefits you and those around you. Remember, again, there is no right or wrong; there is just a practice, and in this instance, there is no practice making perfect.

3: Granting Grace and Loving-Kindness

As you grow in your awareness and attention to your thoughts, your breath, and your being, you will, as research has shown[39] be more attuned to your own needs. You will be in a place to take the time to respond rather than react and to suspend judgment and increase understanding. And so this is the final action item we suggest. The concept can take many forms of words, loving-kindness, grace, and compassion, but the overall meaning is to understand that we are all in this life together. We are all connected, and extending that loving-kindness to ourselves allows us to extend it to others.

In our "never enough" culture, as you pay attention to your thoughts, you may find out that you are quite hard on yourself or hard on others. What would it be like to not fight with yourself inside your own head? What would it be like to not be angry at others? What would it be like to hold others in a compassionate light? These steps can help us extend our sense of mindfulness into our relationships and truly benefit those around us. So what does this look like in your own life?

Pick a day, pick strangers, or pick a family member or friend. But you will want to be intentional about this practice. Notice your thoughts and interactions with this person, and choose thoughts that hold that person in a sense of loving kindness. Slow down, notice your thoughts, breathe, and before you react to this person, remember that they are impermanent, that they too will be gone from this earth one day, as will you, and treat them in a way that honors the truth of this impermanence. An additional suggestion might be to spend a day or many days, eventually every day, giving yourself that same loving-kindness—that same grace. Treat yourself in the same loving way you wished to be treated or were treated as a child, and be present with yourself in those moments, fully being in that experience. While it may be easier to think about being compassionate or kind to others first, the little secret is that it is easier to give something that you already have the capacity for by practicing it with yourself first.

CONCLUSION

This chapter is just a small sampling of information on mindfulness and its benefits. You will find a list of some helpful resources below of scholars who have worked with mindfulness for years. We hope it is a beginning or a reintroduction for you of reasons why this sometimes-ambiguous-sounding practice can be brought into your life and the lives of those you love. It is not something "other" people do, it is something we can all access. While some people do carve out a formal time of the day to practice mindfulness meditation, remember that mindfulness can be done in the same time that you already have, driving to work, folding laundry, mowing the yard, and so forth. The change can be felt in how you approach these tasks and how you approach those moments with your loved ones. Are you fully present in that moment? Are you working toward treating yourself and others with loving-kindness? Are you accepting of the moment as it is and then able to fully respond in the best way possible to that moment? And remember, this is all a process; there is no goal really, just to keep putting one foot in front of the other and living moment to moment.

NOTES

1. John O'Donohue, "Fluent" in Conamara Blues (New York: Harper Perennial, 2004).

2. J. Kabat-Zinn, *Full Catastrophe Living* (New York: Delta Trade Paperbacks, 2009).

3. J. M. Williams and J. Kabat-Zinn, "Mindfulness: Diverse perspectives on its meaning, origins, and multiple applications at the intersection of science and dharma," *Contemporary Buddhism: An Interdisciplinary Journal* 12, no. 1, (2011): 1–18, doi: 10.1080/14639947.2011.564811.

4. B. Bodhi, "What does mindfulness really mean? A canonical perspective," *Contemporary Buddhism: An Interdisciplinary Journal* 12, no. 1 (2011): 19–39, doi: 10.1080/14639947.2011.564813.

5. Williams and Kabat-Zinn, "Mindfulness," 1–18.

6. K. Race, *Mindful Parenting: Simple and Powerful Solutions for Raising Creative, Engaged, Happy Kids in Today's Hectic World* (New York: St. Martin's Griffin, 2014).

7. S. Albers, *Eating mindfully: How to end mindless eating and enjoy a balanced relationship with food*, 2nd ed. (Oakland, CA: New Harbinger Publications, 2012).

8. V. Burch and D. Penman, *You Are Not Your Pain: Using Mindfulness to Relieve Pain, Reduce Stress, and Restore Well-Being* (New York, NY: Flatiron Books, 2013).

9. J. Kabat-Zinn, *Full Catastrophe Living*.

10. Ibid.

11. R. D. Siegel, *The Mindfulness Solution: Everyday Practices for Everyday Problems* (New York: Guilford Press, 2009).

12. Bodhi, "What does mindfulness really mean? A canonical perspective."

13. Williams and Kabat-Zinn, "Mindfulness," 1–18.

14. Kabat-Zinn. *Full Catastrophe Living*.

15. National Institute of Mental Health [NIMH], 2012.

16. Kabat-Zinn. *Full Catastrophe Living*, 6.

17. A. Keane, "The influence of therapist mindfulness practice on psychotherapeutic work: A mixed-methods study," *Mindfulness* 5 (2014): 689–703, doi: 10.1007/s12671-013-02239.

18. Kabat-Zinn. *Full Catastrophe Living*.

19. M. McLeod, ed. and Thich Nhat Hanh, *Your True Home: The Everyday Wisdom of Thich Nhat Hanh* (Boulder, CO: Shambhala, 2011).

20. J. D. Teasdale and M. Chaskalson, "How does mindfulness transform suffering? II: The transformation of dukkha," *Contemporary Buddhism: An Interdisciplinary Journal* 12 (2011): 103–124, doi: 10.1080/14639947.2011.564826.

21. William Shakespeare, *Hamlet*, 2.2, accessed October 20, 2015, http://shakespeare.mit.edu/hamlet/hamlet.2.2.html.

22. Kabat-Zinn. *Full Catastrophe Living.*

23. Ibid.

24. Ibid.

25. C. Feldman and W. Kuyken, "Compassion in the landscape of suffering," *Contemporary Buddhism: An Interdisciplinary Journal* 12, no. 1 (2011): 143–55, doi: 10.1080/14639947.2011.564831.

26. J. D. Teasdale and M. Chaskalson, "How does mindfulness transform suffering? II: The transformation of dukkha," *Contemporary Buddhism: An Interdisciplinary Journal* 12 (2011): 103–24, doi: 10.1080/14639947.2011.564826.

27. Teasdale and Chaskalson, "How does mindfulness transform suffering?"

28. L. M. Monteiro, R. F. Musten, and J. Compson, "Traditional and contemporary mindfulness: Finding the middle path in the tangle of concerns," *Mindfulness* 6 (2014): 1–13, doi: 10.1007/s12671-014-0301-7.

29. Siegel, *The Mindfulness Solution.*

30. S. Barnes et al., "The role of mindfulness in romantic relationship satisfaction and response to relationship stress," *Journal of Marital and Family Therapy* 33, no. 4 (2007): 482–500.

31. J. Carson et al., "Mindfulness-Based Relationship Enhancement," *Behavior Therapy* 35 (2004): 471–94.

32. Siegel, *The Mindfulness Solution.*

33. T. N. Hanh, *Present Moment Wonderful Moment: Mindfulness Verses for Daily Living* (Berkley, CA: Parallax Press, 2006), 163.

34. Bodhi, "What does mindfulness really mean? A canonical perspective."

35. Kabat-Zinn. *Full Catastrophe Living.*

36. T. N. Hanh, *Present Moment Wonderful Moment.*

37. Kabat-Zinn. *Full Catastrophe Living*, 13.

38. T. N. Hanh, *Present Moment Wonderful Moment.*

39. A. Keane, "The influence of therapist mindfulness practice on psychotherapeutic work."

SECTION

3

OUR BODIES

*"Take care of your body. It's the
only place you have to live."*

—*Jim Rohn*

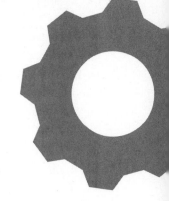
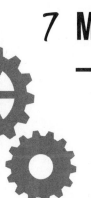

7 MAKE PEACE WITH FOOD —AND YOURSELF

BY EMILY FONNESBECK, RD

"ONE CANNOT THINK WELL, LOVE WELL, SLEEP WELL, IF
ONE HAS NOT DINED WELL."[1] —VIRGINIA WOOLF

EMILY FONNESBECK, RD, *received her degree at Brigham Young University. She is a member of the Academy of Nutrition and Dietetics and belongs to the practice groups of Behavioral Health Nutrition and Sports, Cardiovascular, and Wellness Nutrition. She has completed training in adult weight management and is a certified LEAP therapist, specializing in delayed food sensitivity reactions typically associated with autoimmune, digestive, and inflammatory conditions. Emily has a passion for nutrition. She loves creating flavorful and healthy meals for her family to enjoy. She takes great pleasure in cooking for family and friends and loves the satisfaction of coming together to enjoy a meal. As a family, they enjoy being outdoors in the water or the mountains. She appreciates staying active through yoga, biking, running, and weight training.*

INTRODUCTION

When I first started my professional career, I truly believed that a lack of knowledge about food was the reason behind poor food choices. As I taught group classes and counseled individuals privately, I focused my energy on telling people what to eat. I soon realized that I wasn't at all helpful or inspiring. This left me discouraged, and I questioned my ability to truly help others. As a result, I decided to quit talking and start listening. What I learned was that we all know what to eat. If two plates were put in front of any of us and we were told to take the healthier choice, we would all make the "correct" choice. Instead of asking *what* you eat, a far better question is *why* you eat. Food choices are a blend of physiological and psychological needs, influenced greatly by how you feel about yourself.

Unfortunately, it's easy to feel unvalued and inferior when you don't live up to the ideal standard of beauty, fitness, and health that society has painted (whether male or female). I would like to challenge that ideal and help you understand the damage that can come to physical, emotional, and mental health by not accepting yourself as unique, special, and worthy of love—most important self-love. I would also like to offer some nutrition tools to help you on your own road to understanding, loving, and taking care of your body.

SELF-ACCEPTANCE

I believe there is a natural yearning we all have to improve and be just a little bit better. Many individuals I work with want just that, and I find it completely inspiring! I would encourage you to go with that feeling, but I would like to offer a suggestion. *In terms of food and health, I would recommend ditching numbers or rigid, tight controls and engage in self-care.* Self-care feels good. It builds a more positive body image, makes us less susceptible to stress and anxiety, improves immunity, increases positive thinking, and leads to patience and compassion for yourself and others. Self-care can feel self-indulgent or selfish to some, but I believe the exact opposite. We are only able to serve others when we have something to give. If we neglect our own needs, we risk deep levels of unhappiness, low self-esteem, resentment, and feeling burned out.

The great paradox that exists in health is this: being encouraged to live up to society's unrealistic idea of health in order to improve your own health but feeling like a failure for not being able to do so almost always leads to giving up and not trying at all. It's time for a different approach! Health can come right now. In fact, right now is the only time you really have to make an impact on your health. Trying to control an outcome is futile, but focusing on what is right in front of you and loving yourself enough to take care of yourself will allow you to make choices that are in your best interest.

The idea of self-love can feel impossible. If that feels like a stretch for now, I would encourage you to find self-acceptance. Accepting something doesn't mean you have to love it; it means that you are willing to be honest and truthful about where you are, how you got there, and where you would like to go. It allows you to see things as they really are—what is working and what isn't. For many, acceptance means stagnation, or if I accept myself, then I won't be able to change. In reality, the opposite is actually true. Take a look at this cycle of non-acceptance:[2]

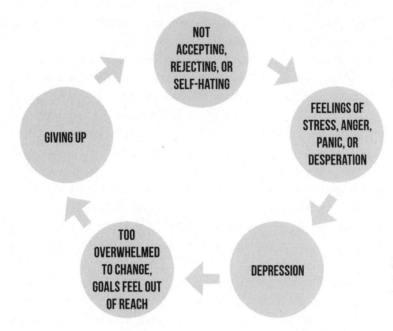

If you reject or hate your body, it can lead to emotional distress at best and mental illness at worst. This leads you to feel overwhelmed, discouraged, and hopeless. On the other hand, look what happens when you accept yourself, your body, and your situation:

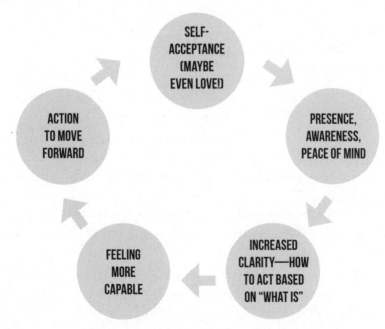

Self-acceptance (and self-love if you can!) leads to being present and aware of what's happening in and around you right now. This peace of mind allows for clarity on how to act and invites inspiration and direction for how to handle the situation. The reward is feeling capable to move forward and act in ways that facilitate change. You are able to make decisions that are in your best interest.

It's expected and natural to bounce around from cycle to cycle as you move forward. The key is to remember that you *can* accept yourself. You are worthy of love and care no matter what's happened in the past, where you are right now, what your situation, or how far you may or may not be from your goal. Again, all you have is right now. You are worth more than you give yourself credit for, and you—more than anyone else—deserve your own love, care, and acceptance. You came to this world in the body you were meant to. You were given your own set of gifts, experiences, challenges, and victories. If we take a look around, we realize that we all come in different shapes and sizes, with unique personalities, wisdom, and gifts to share. What a boring world we would live in if we all looked and behaved the same. To help you find self-acceptance, I would like to advocate for the idea of Health at Every Size.

HEALTH AT EVERY SIZE

If we look at the data, we do in fact see that health comes at every size. Dr. Linda Bacon, author of *Health at Every Size* (HAES), states, "Fat isn't the problem. Dieting is the problem. A society that rejects anyone whose body shape or size doesn't match an impossible ideal is the problem. A medical establishment that equates 'thin' with 'healthy' is the problem."[3] In this same book, she outlines research to support the following:

1. There is no clear evidence that people with "normal" weight actually live longer than people who are "overweight," and many epidemiologic studies actually show "overweight" individuals living as long or longer.

2. Studies on the health risks associated with weight rarely will account for fitness levels, physical activity, nutrient intake, weight cycling, or socioeconomic status. All of these factors play a role in health, and when studies do control for these factors, risk of disease—regardless of weight—is reduced or disappears. When healthy behaviors are present, disease risk decreases as well as the risk of unhealthy weight gain.

3. There has been no study to show that weight loss increases life expectancy. However, there are many studies that indicate intentional weight loss may increase the risk of dying early from certain diseases.

It appears as though maintaining, not gaining or losing, is the better solution. While there are, indeed, exceptions to every rule, there needs to be a more balanced approach and message about weight instead of the single story we believe about it.[4]

Do me a favor and close your eyes. Imagine waking up tomorrow morning to a world that is free of labels and judgment. You find a safe environment where love and acceptance abound. What would you do differently? Do you feel you would have more confidence? Do you think you would find it easier to be who you really are? Would you find it easier to share your thoughts and feelings with others? Or be happy to be you?

I would hope you understand this: you have the ability to create that world inside of you. By loving and accepting yourself unconditionally, you allow others to do the same. Each of us perpetuates the problem daily by not loving ourselves to the fullest. When you love yourself unconditionally, you are better able to love others unconditionally. It starts with you. If we want to make a difference and create environments that are safe, it has to start with us identifying our own weight biases and replacing them with love and acceptance.

In order to help you do that, I would like to list the principles of Health at Every Size along with a quote from the book of the same name:

> Let's face facts. We've lost the war on obesity. Fighting fat hasn't made the fat go away. And being thinner, even if we knew how to successfully accomplish it, will not necessarily make us healthier or happier. The war on obesity has taken its toll. Extensive "collateral damage" has resulted: Food and body preoccupation, self-hatred, eating disorders, discrimination, poor health. . . . Few of us are at peace with our bodies, whether because we're fat or because we fear becoming fat. Health at Every Size is the new peace movement. Very simply, it acknowledges that good health can best be realized independent from considerations of size. It supports people—of all sizes—in addressing health directly by adopting healthy behaviors.[5]

I wholeheartedly agree and have seen this movement have a dramatic impact on those that I work with. By loving and accepting the body you are in, you will want to treat it well. By engaging in self-care practices, you can find health at any size. Your body will find its healthy weight when it is listened to, trusted, and cared for.

Health at Every Size encourages the following:[6]

1. Accepting and respecting the natural diversity of body sizes and shapes.

2. Eating in a flexible manner that values pleasure and honors internal cues of hunger, satiety, and appetite.

3. Finding the joy in moving one's body and becoming more physically vital.

This is how you can participate in the HAES movement, and I quote the HAES association here:[7]

1. Accept your size. Love and appreciate the body you have. Self-acceptance empowers you to move on and make positive changes.

2. Trust yourself. We all have internal systems designed to keep us healthy—and at a healthy weight. Support your body in naturally finding its appropriate weight by honoring its signals of hunger, fullness, and appetite.

3. Adopt healthy lifestyle habits.

Develop and nurture connections with others and look for purpose and meaning in your life. Fulfilling your social, emotional, and spiritual needs restores food to its rightful place as a source of nourishment and pleasure.

• Find the joy in moving your body and becoming more physically vital in your everyday life.

• Eat when you're hungry, stop when you're full, and seek out pleasurable and satisfying foods.

• Tailor your tastes so that you enjoy more nutritious foods, staying mindful that there is plenty of room for less nutritious choices in the context of an overall healthy diet and lifestyle.

4. Embrace size diversity. Humans come in a variety of sizes and shapes. Be open to the beauty found across the spectrum, and support others in recognizing their unique attractiveness.

Health and wellness is much bigger than what foods you do and don't eat. Diets or rigid food rules can cause anxiety and stress, which is counterproductive to health. Don't let the desire to lose weight make you lose sight of the bigger picture. While weight loss may be helpful for some, adopting healthier behaviors as a part of self-care will allow for possible needed changes in weight. Ultimately, health is a product of healthy behaviors and is not determined by weight.

SELF-CARE

There is nothing more freeing than not needing outside validation for who you are. Once you accept yourself and the fact that you don't need to meet an impossible ideal, you are free to take care of yourself. What does self-care look like? That might depend on the individual. But here are common positive behaviors, most of which will be discussed here or in other chapters.

1. Adequate sleep. Research shows us the magic number is anywhere between seven to nine hours, with most of us getting much less. Sleep is when your body heals and repairs itself. It needs that time to recover and be ready for another day. Establishing a night routine by turning off electronics, relaxing your mind and getting to bed a little earlier can pay off exponentially.[8]

2. Physical activity. Our bodies are designed to move. They crave it, actually. Movement brings a release, invites creativity, and enhances mood. Physical activity doesn't have to mean tortuous exercise, it just means moving your body in a way you enjoy. The sweet spot for exercise appears to be thirty minutes, with longer sessions being up to you! You can even do it in three ten-minute sessions if you need to.[9] Short workouts can actually boost hormone balance and endocrine function as well as give the immune system a kick-start.[10, 11]

• If you have a desk job and are sitting most of the day, try setting a timer to remind you to take a five- to ten-minute stretch and walk break each hour. If you are a parent home with children during the day, find ways to be active with them and make it a family affair.

3. Stress reduction. Stress—we all have it. The key is to learn how to manage it effectively before it manages you. Setting emotional boundaries in relationships, saying no when you need to, learning deep breathing techniques, participating in meditation, making time for exercise, getting a massage . . . find an effective strategy for you! Work to bring awareness to stress and how it feels to you, and you will be able to identify and adapt before it gets out of hand.

4. Set a flexible structure. Establishing a somewhat regular routine can help you feel empowered and accomplished. In terms of food, I would recommend three regular, well-balanced meals with snacks between, depending on your hunger levels. Balanced meals include fruits, vegetables, complex carbohydrates, lean proteins and healthy fats.

- I don't think it is a coincidence that our body chemistry is designed to eat regularly throughout the day. It serves as a great reminder to take a break from life every three to four hours to sit and engage in self-care by nourishing and fueling our minds and bodies.

It is this last item on which I would like to expand. As you accept where you are and move forward in productive change, nutrition information becomes a tool rather than a weapon. The following information is meant to be just that—tools for your own personal growth.

FINDING NUTRITIONAL BALANCE

The most common solution for changing food behavior is to start a diet. It is estimated that forty-five million Americans diet each year, making the weight loss market a $33-billion industry annually. However, 95 percent of diets fail, and most will likely regain the weight lost within one to five years.[12] Weight regain typically occurs right after a period of dieting ends, and researchers believe this is due to an energy gap—calorie restriction or caloric deficit—created when dieting. When expending more energy than you are taking in, there is a physiological drive to eat, or a hyperphagic response, when allowed to eat without restriction.[13] Basically, research shows dieting results in weight loss, but long-term maintenance is unlikely due to the fact that you are working against your basic physiological function, or as I like to call it—being at war with yourself. It's been said that "insanity is repeating the same mistakes and expecting different results."[14] Dieting, calorie counting, and obsessively thinking about food and how to control both our diets and our impulse to eat is getting us nowhere. It's also a miserable way to live, with large ramifications for physical and emotional health. While the research is still unclear, gaining and losing weight over and over, also known as "yo-yo dieting," may affect body composition, favoring greater fat mass in some conditions.[15, 16] Weight cycling also appears to increase risk for life dissatisfaction, binge eating and mental illness.[17]

Extremes are easy, and we often find ourselves bouncing back and forth between rigidity (diets) and chaos. In my experience, restriction breeds rebellion, and the level of rigidity is directly correlated with the level of resulting chaos. Extreme rigidity = extreme chaos. Here's the cycle:

1. Start a diet with strict rules.

2. Experience boredom and feelings of deprivation from lack of variety.

3. Break strict dietary rules and "cheat" on diet.

4. Feel guilty for "cheating," and give up altogether.

5. Eat all the foods you weren't allowed on the diet.

And then it starts over again. In his book *The Mindful Therapist*, Dr. Dan Siegel describes mental health as balance between rigidity and chaos.[18] That has always stuck with me. If our thoughts are rigid or chaotic, then our behaviors will also be. Balanced thoughts are nonjudgmental and are open to all possibilities. If we can find balance in our thinking, we can find balance in behavior. The key, then, is to change how you think about food. Assigning moral character to food, having lists of good and bad foods, and villainizing certain foods or food groups will never result in a healthy relationship with food. Being present and open to all possibilities means accepting food without judgment. I realize this sounds scary, especially with all the nutrition noise we are bombarded with every day. However, food shouldn't hold power over you. It's time you take your power back by making peace with it.

Let's face it, food has a huge impact on our health. However, in the nutrition culture we live in, food and nutrition becomes confusing, frustrating, and overwhelming, and then we just want to throw in the towel. The confusion and fearmongering that is so abundant prevents us from seeing things as they really are. When we see nutrition for what it is, in all its glorious simplicity, we can use it to our benefit in order to meet our health and wellness goals. There are basic principles of nutrition that, if applied, can have huge impacts on our health. The following discussion is meant to give guidance for those seeking understanding of nutrition amid so many trends and ideas. I hope you don't misunderstand my intention with using calories as part of this discussion. While I don't recommend counting calories, because it tends to lead to a diet mentality, they are a currency most people relate to and understand. I would like to use them here only to illustrate the inverse relationship between nutrient density and calorie density—principles that can give you an idea for how to increase the overall nutrient density of each of your meals, without counting calories

NUTRIENT DENSITY VERSUS CALORIE DENSITY

There are two types of receptors in your stomach: stretch receptors and density receptors. Both of these play a large role in helping you feel full and satisfied from your meals. The goal then would be to trigger both of them in order to get the most out of your meals. Stretch receptors, as you could probably guess, sense stomach stretch. As you chew your food and swallow it, food goes to your stomach, the stomach is stretched, and these receptors send hormones to your brain, signaling that you are eating and getting full.

A high-volume meal is key to triggering these receptors, but the trick is to trigger them with foods that are nutrient-dense rather than calorie-dense. As an experienced eater, you recognize that this is a large part of satisfaction! Before you ever start eating, you want to look at your plate and feel that there is enough food. Therefore, volume contributes greatly to both physiological and psychological satisfaction.[19, 20] You can see this demonstrated in the image below (adapted from DiseaseProof.com):

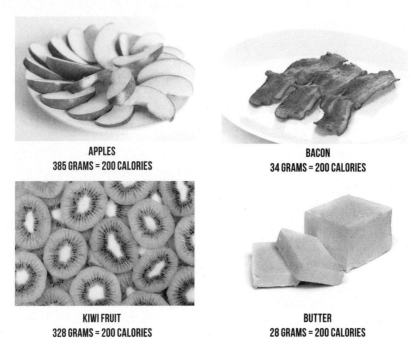

APPLES
385 GRAMS = 200 CALORIES

BACON
34 GRAMS = 200 CALORIES

KIWI FRUIT
328 GRAMS = 200 CALORIES

BUTTER
28 GRAMS = 200 CALORIES

Research reveals that each of us eats about the same amount of food per day—about three to five pounds by weight on average. Obviously this varies depending on size, gender, and activity level, with some individuals needing less than three and some individuals needing more than five. But taking that average will help us compare nutrient density and calorie density.[21]

Foods that are high in volume are foods high in water and fiber content. These foods are nutrient-dense, or high in nutrition when we compare calories per pound. Since we average three to five pounds of food each day, increasing the nutrient density per pound and decreasing the calorie density per pound can help us manage our weight. In addition, foods high in nutrient density will be as they sound—high in vitamins, minerals, antioxidants, phytochemicals, fiber and water—high in nutrition. These compounds are what heal and repair the body from oxidative damage and inflammation, therefore preventing or treating chronic diseases such as diabetes, heart disease and the like. Let's take a look at the different food groups and were they fall in terms of nutrient density versus calorie density:[22, 23]

- vegetables = 100 calories per pound

- fruit = 300 calories per pound

- whole, intact grains and starchy vegetables = 500 calories per pound (brown rice, oats, wheat, barley, spelt, quinoa, corn, potatoes, sweet potatoes, butternut squash, acorn squash, and so on)

- beans = 600 calories per pound

- animal products = 1,000 calories per pound (dairy products, eggs, meat, fish, poultry—a large variety, and this is an average)

- processed complex carbohydrates = 1,400 calories per pound (whole grain breads, whole grain crackers, whole grain cereals, and so on)

- processed, packaged foods = 2,300 calories per pound

- nuts and seeds = 2,800 calories per pound (avocado is included here)

- oils and fats = 4,000 calories per pound

If you were to eat four pounds of vegetables, you would eat four hundred calories. It's pretty hard to overeat on vegetables, because they are high in fiber and water, which easily signals our stretch receptors for fullness. But can you eat a plate of vegetables and feel satisfied? This is not a trick question. The answer is no! If you'll remember, there is a second type of receptor called density receptors. These receptors are there to ensure survival and sense the caloric density of a meal. Eating only four hundred calories a day wouldn't get you very far, so these receptors are there to make sure you eat enough.

Moving up this scale, fruit is three hundred calories per pound. By making an effort to add a fruit or vegetable each time you eat, you dramatically increase nutrient density. This simple addition will likely help you feel more full and satisfied, deliver important nutrients to your body, and possibly take the place of other, less nutrient-dense food choices.

Whole, intact grains means that the grain is as it appears just out of the ground, before processing or grinding in any way. Examples include brown rice, oats, wheat berries (the whole kernel of wheat before it's ground to flour), barley, bulgur, and so on. Whole grain pasta would also be included, due the fact that when it's cooked, it absorbs water and expands.

A bit further down the list you see processed complex carbohydrates, which begs explaining at this point. This category is for whole grain breads, whole grain cereals, and whole grain crackers. While they are a whole grain, they will be more calorie-dense. One cup of cooked brown rice (a whole, intact grain) is two hundred calories, while one cup of whole grain flour is close to four to five hundred calories. See the difference?

I don't wish to bad-mouth any of these food groups (remember, a healthy relationship with food means avoiding assignment of moral character!) and whole grain breads can be a great, convenient, and healthy choice. With all the confusion about bread, let's see things as they are. If I had whole grain toast with breakfast, a sandwich for lunch (made with two slices of whole grain bread) and a whole grain roll with dinner, my overall calorie density would be greater than if I had a piece of whole grain toast for breakfast, brown rice for lunch, and a sweet potato for dinner. The lesson learned here is to aim for variety.

Beans have six hundred calories per pound, and I dare anyone to eat four pounds of beans and want to live to tell about it. Enough said.

Therein lies the key: the amount of fiber and water inherent in these first four food groups helps to signal fullness. In order to satisfy both types of receptors while keeping nutrient density high, I recommend using this plate method for an eight-inch plate:

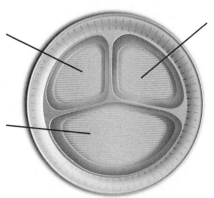

LEAN PROTEINS

Meat, poultry, fish, game, eggs, beans, legumes, nuts, seeds, dairy products, and soy (tofu, tempeh, edamame, and soy milk).

VEGETABLES & FRUITS

Any! Try to eat a good variety and opt for fresh or frozen more often than canned, dried, or juiced.

COMPLEX CARBOHYDRATES

Oats, brown rice, barley, bulgur, wheat, rye, spelt, quinoa, kamut, millet, buckwheat, teff, sorghum, amaranth, corn, potatoes, sweet potatoes, butternut squash, acorn squash, beans. (Try to make at least half of your grains each day whole grains.)

HEALTHY FATS: *Although not included in the visual, it is important to cook and prepare meals with healthy fats. Fat is often forgotten when trying to control calories, but it is also essential to feeling satisfied from meals, not to mention for maintaining good health. Try using olive, coconut, nuts, seeds, avocado, and even a little butter. Other ways to include fats in your meals may come from the food choices themselves, such as fatty fish (salmon, tuna, herring, trout, mackerel, sardines, and so on), egg yolks, dairy, and meat products.*

Basically, aim to make one-half to three-quarters of your plate from the first four food groups, using the remaining food groups as flavor enhancers, for texture, and for garnish. This will satisfy your need for volume, as well as your need to move up the scale in calorie density to trigger density receptors. This will allow for a big-picture approach to food and prevents the need to get nit picky. Foods that are often villainized become less of an issue when you approach them in a balanced way. What matters most is what you are doing most of the time, consistently making your plate look like this. It matters less if you use a bit of butter on your vegetables when half of your plate is full of them. It matters less if you choose to have a fluffy white roll with dinner when it's a quarter of your plate and that plate includes a lean protein and fruits and vegetables. It matters less if you choose to have pizza for dinner when you balance it with a high-nutrient-dense salad that takes up half your plate. Basically, all foods can fit when consumed in balance. Aim for consistency and keep a "big picture" approach. It will keep you sane!

With this approach, 75 percent of your plate is coming from the ground and is high in fiber and nutrition. In the research it's called a plant-based diet, and we have great data on the health benefits of this approach.

> Studies exploring the risk of overweight and food groups and dietary patterns indicate that a plant-based diet seems to be a sensible approach for the prevention of obesity in children. Plant-based diets are low in energy density and high in complex carbohydrate, fiber, and water, which may increase satiety and resting energy expenditure. . . .
>
> [Plant-based diets] caused more calories to be burned after meals, in contrast to [non-plant-based diets,] which may cause fewer calories to be burned because food is being stored as fat. . . .
>
> The future of health care will involve an evolution toward a paradigm where the prevention and treatment of disease is centered, not on a pill or surgical procedure, but on another serving of fruits and vegetables. . . .
>
> Plant-based eating may successfully control weight, prevent and treat type II diabetes, help prevent an abdominal aortic aneurysm, prevent gallstones, improve cognition, prevent age related macular degeneration, cataracts, slow aging, raise childhood IQ, improve body-odor, reduce waist circumference, reduce allergies, reduce abdominal fat, and cut down on the need for drugs and surgery. Plant-based diets are also beneficial for the prevention and treatment of rheumatoid arthritis, erectile dysfunction, and diabetes.[24]

I believe this data speaks to our ability to work with our body's natural chemistry rather than against it. Instead of dieting and counting calories (being at war with yourself), eating nutrient-dense meals (based on the plate method) can actually increase your metabolic rate and will help you feel full and satisfied while contributing to weight and chronic disease management (letting your head and your body be on the same team).

FLEXIBLE STRUCTURE

When you have felt chaotic with food, it's natural to want a rigid plan to put as much space between you and the problematic behavior as possible, and understandably so. It is also natural to feel a complete lack of trust with yourself and your ability to make decisions that are in your best interest. But as you can see, you don't want a diet. What you want is a plan, a flexible plan, which allows you to both meet your health and wellness goals and stay sane in the process. A flexible structure is what I classify as the balance between rigidity and chaos. Use a flexible rather than a rigid set of rules and a structure rather than chaos, because having no boundaries with food isn't healthy either. Based on the principles of nutrient density versus calorie density and the basic guidelines found in the plate method, I would invite you to do the following:

1. Eat balanced meals, using the plate method, every three to four hours, adding snacks as needed based on meal timing and hunger.

2. Focus on consistency not perfection, and keep a big-picture perspective that allows you to include your favorite "deal breakers."

3. Slow down and enjoy your meal for physiological and psychological satisfaction, and bring awareness to judgments that come up about yourself or the food as you eat.

I would like to expand on each of these three recommendations.

EAT BALANCED MEALS

When it comes to food, the most important self-care technique would be eating regular, balanced meals. Our bodies crave rhythm and structure. We are cyclical creatures! Think about it—we have sleep cycles, hormonal cycles, digestion rhythms, and life cycles. Additionally, the earth circles the sun, there are day and night cycles . . . we could go on and on! Our digestive rhythms require regular balanced meals. Skipping meals can often cause bloating, gas, indigestion and diarrhea, or constipation, while regular, balanced meals can aid in the natural contractions that break down foods for absorption and move waste through. Regular eating times can prevent getting overly hungry and subsequent overeating. Because our digestive tracts can only handle so much food at one time, overeating causes stress on our body and its ability to make adequate digestive enzymes and hormones (including insulin and appetite-regulating hormones, to name a few) to keep up with the amount of food eaten. The result would be inflammation and metabolic changes that could lead to chronic diseases such as diabetes, high blood pressure, high cholesterol, and heart disease.

I don't think it's a coincidence that we are designed to need nourishment every three to five hours. It serves as a great reminder to take a break from life regularly throughout the day to engage in self-care practices. By allowing yourself to take breaks three times a day, if just for ten to twenty minutes, you will be more productive. I'm sure any of us can think of times when we went too long without food and became foggy-headed, irritable, short-tempered, fatigued and ornery—or "hangry" as we like to call it at our house, meaning hungry-angry. Taking time for yourself is not selfish. In fact, self-care is probably the most unselfish thing you can do. You can fill someone else's cup only if your cup is full. By taking care of you, you are better able to help and serve others and be what you need to be for coworkers, friends, or family members.

FOCUS ON CONSISTENCY INSTEAD OF PERFECTION

I do believe the key to maintaining a flexible structure is to plan ahead and keep it simple. It has been observed that Albert Einstein wore the same outfit every day.[16] Those who claim this say he did it to save brainpower. I really have no idea if it's true, but I think it's a pretty powerful concept. How much time, energy, and anxiety do you use in making decisions each day? Before you even leave the house you have probably had to choose what to wear, if and when to exercise, what to eat for meals, what do with your children, and how to handle situations at work. We make dozens of decisions, and it's exhausting! In my experience, the fewer choices you have to make, the easier life is. There are plenty of decisions you can't opt out on, but I do feel there are many areas of your life you can streamline, minimize, and simplify. Food choices are definitely one of those. If your food choices and food preparation give you anxiety or take up too much of your precious time, you aren't doing it right. Eating healthy will always take effort, but it shouldn't be stressful or take the place of more important things. I would recommend planning two to four breakfasts, two to four lunches, and two to four snacks that can be rotated throughout the week. For dinner, you would probably benefit from planning at least five dinners, with one night to be used as leftovers and one night out (to be realistic). Paste meal and snack ideas on the refrigerator. Shop for ingredients for each of those meals so your kitchen is stocked. Then as you go throughout the week, you will find meal assembly a breeze. Feel free to repeat that same meal plan from week to week, adding new recipes as often as you choose for variety without being overwhelmed with too many options. With a couple hours of food planning, shopping, and simple food prep on the weekend, you won't have to think much about food during the week. This is perfect, given you have way more important things to do with your time!

Here are lists of examples for complex carbohydrates, protein choices, and added fats:

Complex Carbohydrates

Oats, brown rice, barley, bulgur, wheat, rye, spelt, quinoa, kamut, millet, buckwheat, teff, sorghum, amaranth, corn, potatoes, sweet potatoes, butternut squash, acorn squash, and beans.

Lean Proteins

Beans (they can be both a protein and a carbohydrate), meat, poultry, fish, eggs, dairy products, soy products, nuts, and seeds.

Fats

Oils, avocado, butter, gravies, and dressings.

Here are some ideas to get you thinking:

Breakfast

- whole grain bread with peanut butter and bananas
- oatmeal topped with nuts and fruit
- egg, bean, and vegetable scramble
- scrambled eggs, roasted potatoes, and fruit
- smoothie or parfait with fruit, yogurt, and nuts or granola

Lunch

- brown rice, beans, and vegetables with salsa and guacamole
- turkey sandwich with carrot and vegetable sticks dipped in hummus
- vegetable bean soup with whole grain crackers
- sweet potato topped with chicken, vegetables, and avocado
- cottage cheese with veggie sticks and whole grain pita

Dinner

- salmon with brown rice and vegetables
- chili and baked potato topped with avocado
- whole grain pasta with vegetables, ground beef, and marinara sauce
- lentil vegetable soup
- chicken with sweet potato fries and vegetables

It's always interesting to me how taken aback individuals are when I list ideas like this. Many times I hear, "You mean, I can eat bread?" or "It's okay to eat avocado?" or "Potatoes don't have too many carbs?" I understand where these questions are coming from, and it's usually from the diet mentality. The decade you are in when you decide to diet would dictate what macronutrient to be afraid of. Fat-free diets were used predominately in the 1990s, whereas fat is now considered to be a dieter's friend and carbohydrates are shunned. In my experience, inadequate fat *and* carbohydrates at each meal is often what leads to overeating and bingeing. Eating meals that are satisfying and filling is exactly what you want to be doing. Otherwise, your meals will leave you unsatisfied and preoccupied with food, leading to poor productivity and eventual binges on restricted foods or restricted macronutrients. Food binges or overeating episodes usually are with high-fat and high-carbohydrate foods. By eliminating either or both (rigidity), you will likely set yourself up for overeating (chaos). Establishing regular meal times that are balanced and satisfying will allow you to move on from meals to focus on much more important aspects of your life! Feeling full and satisfied from your meals isn't the problem; it's the solution. Not feeling satisfied from meals is what leads to problematic behaviors.

Establishing a flexible structure with regular, balanced meals will allow you to take care of yourself. As I mentioned, taking a break from life to nourish yourself can help you feel valued and taken care of. This will help you avoid feeling the need to use food as a reward in the afternoon or late evening (the most common times for food rewards), since you are letting it nourish you all day. More effective coping strategies for stress can then take its place. As you eat, slow down and really savor your food. Feeling physiologically and psychologically satisfied from your meal is essential to improving your relationship with food. Up until this point, you may have felt that food was the enemy, and it may have been a source of anxiety or stress for you. I hope moving forward you can see that food is your friend and that you have every right to enjoy it and feel satisfied from it. There are many pleasures in life—food being one of them. Don't be afraid to enjoy it!

SLOW DOWN AND ENJOY MEALS

As you eat your meals, focus on hunger and fullness cues. We often eat based on external cues such as food availability, time of day, or calorie allotment. As you set regular meal times with balanced meals, you are better able to tune into your own internal signals of hunger and fullness. Remember: you were born as an intuitive eater. We lose the ability to hear those signals only because we quit practicing. It's not about learning something new; it's about uncovering what you already have. When you do this, you see that you have been able to trust yourself with food all along—no diet needed. Interestingly enough, studies have shown that individuals who are preoccupied with their appearance are less likely to listen to their body cues. This would be another benefit of self-acceptance and self-care.[26] To help you start practicing, you can refer to this hunger scale:

10	Painfully full and may feel sick.
9	Stuffed and uncomfortable.
8	Full. You don't want anything else to eat.
7	Totally satisfied. Hunger gone for a few hours.
6	Satisfied but could easily eat more.
5	Neither hungry nor full. Neutral.
4	Hungry. It's time to think about what to eat.
3	Stomach growling. Have hunger pains.
2	Preoccupied with hunger. All food looks good.
1	So hungry you will eat anything.

Looking at this scale, you would be wise to stay within the range of four to seven. Below a four, food becomes hyperpalatable, meaning it tastes even better and is much more appealing. You've probably been at a three or below, where anything sounds good. You can stay much more levelheaded about food choices when making the decision at a four rather than a one. If you are eating consistent, balanced meals, this will be easy to do. On the opposite end, it might take some practice for you to know what "being satisfied, with your hunger gone for a few hours" feels like. Be patient with yourself as you unlearn dieting behaviors and reconnect with your own body wisdom. Repairing relationships take time, nurturing, love, and attention. Your relationship with food and your body will need the same.

However, as you start eating more regularly, you will have more opportunities to practice. I've thought a lot about it, and I don't think there is anything we do as often as eat. As you practice making intentional, purposeful, and mindful decisions in building a meal, while taking time to relax and enjoy without judgment, I think you will be surprised at how that behavior transfers to other areas of your life. You may find yourself being more mindful with decisions while finding it easier to slow down and enjoy the present. The frequency of eating events provides an intense learning process, and you will be able to look back at the week or month or year and see just how far you have come because of how many opportunities you have had to practice.

As an aside, connecting with your body allows you to become your own health expert. For those of you who suffer from certain diseases or food sensitivities, your body will alert you to foods that could causes symptoms. Our bodies are always communicating with us, and as you tune in, you will be able to understand what it is saying. I also recommend working with a trained nutrition professional to help you decipher the messages.

I would also have you know that, in my professional experience, stress and anxiety can have a larger impact in the way food is digested than people realize. The digestive tract is known as "the second brain." What we think in our heads, we feel in our digestive tract. If the stress or anxiety is about the food, then the resulting symptoms may be even more severe. Allowing food to just be what it is rather than assigning moral character or putting unrealistic negative or positive expectations on it is the first step to reducing that anxiety.

EMOTIONAL EATING

We can't talk about physical hunger without talking about emotional hunger, which is a common concern. Typically the conversation around emotional eating focuses on the behavior rather than the origin. The solution then would be to remove the food, calling it anything from a trigger to an addiction. However, the food typically isn't the problem, it's just the way you cope with an emotion. Until you get to the root of the problem, which is to understand and feel the emotional you are wanting to avoid or the emotion that is missing in your life, the problem will remain. Cleaning out your kitchen, putting yourself on a diet, telling yourself "never again" will actually only perpetuate the problem. I'll share some examples.

When you are feeling lonely, you might look for something to fill that void. Many turn to food as a way to turn the ache of loneliness into a physical stomachache from overeating, which often is easier to manage and understand than the actual feeling of empty loneliness. Or maybe you feel like a food addict and are unable to stop eating. There seems to be an insatiable appetite, even without physical signs of hunger. It's likely you may be starving for love, attention, and connection—a basic need for everyone.

We are complex beings with many needs and appetites. Don't sell yourself short! You deserve to have those needs met in health-promoting ways that take care of you! Allowing yourself time to feel, process, identify, and respond in ways that meet your needs is the best thing you can do for yourself. As you allow yourself to feel, you will realize that you feel all feelings more intensely. One of my (many) favorite quotes from shame researcher Brené Brown says, "We cannot selectively numb emotions. When we numb the painful emotions, we also numb the positive emotions."[27] When working with individuals on emotional eating, I like to remind them of that. When you don't allow yourself to feel sad, hurt, frustrated, angry, you won't be able to feel happiness, joy, or peace. The problem isn't that you don't want to feel bad, it's that you don't want to feel anything. Feelings make us vulnerable and can be uncomfortable, but as you become more aware of your feelings—and remember that they are just feelings—you are better able to be present with and accepting of them. You then become better able to be present with other people's emotions and truly connect. Allow yourself to feel; it allows your understanding and compassion to grow! You will also find that life becomes sweeter as your feelings of happiness, gratitude, peace, love, and joy intensify.

Physical Hunger	Emotional Hunger
comes on gradually and can be postponed	comes on suddenly and feels urgent
can be satisfied with any type of food	causes specific cravings, pizza, chocolate, ice cream, and so on
once you're full, you can stop eating	eat more than you normally would and feel uncomfortably full
causes satisfaction, not guilt	leaves you feeling guilty and cross with yourself

This graphic (adapted from www.thelondoner.me) may help you discern between physical hunger and emotional hunger. Physical hunger is actually fairly easy to identify *if* you are eating consistent well-balanced meals as recommended previously. Eating on a more flexible structure will allow your body to return to its natural rhythm. When truly hungry for food, there are many foods you will find appealing. Anything sounds good when you need to eat! Emotional hunger is much more picky, and you usually zero in on one particular food. It's also pretty sudden, especially if you are caught off guard with bad news, frustration in a particular moment, or anger over an event.

Allowing yourself to feel and understand is essential as well as using coping strategies that promote physical, emotional, and mental health rather than detracting from it. Setting proper emotional boundaries with your thoughts and with others is also effective.

I do feel it's important to note that it's impossible not to blur emotional and physical hunger a bit. We are emotional creatures! For example, in the middle of a long, stressful afternoon, you may notice signs of physical hunger. You know you are physically hungry and need to eat, but you also would like to derive pleasure from the food you are eating to feel emotionally and psychologically satisfied. You may decide that tortilla chips and guacamole sound really good, but remembering the principles of nutrient density versus calorie density, you choose to add some salsa, carrot sticks, and apple slices. This would increase the volume and nutrient density of the snack, therefore needing less volume from the more calorie-dense foods chosen. You allow yourself to sit and enjoy your snack as a way to break from the day and relax. You notice signs of fullness as you listen to your body wisdom. Feeling physiologically and psychologically satisfied and refreshed, you find you can finish the day in a productive and levelheaded manner. Food should be pleasurable, and it should enhance your mood, among many other things in your life. There is a big difference between eating for pleasure and eating to numb, and the above example is that of pleasure. Eating to numb may look like a trip to the vending machine for a bag of potato chips that you crunch and bite vigorously in order to avoid biting someone else's head off in anger. While it might not always go as smoothly as the first example, taking care of yourself and understanding how you feel will decrease the likelihood of using food as avoidance.

Patrece's Experience

For the past year and a half, I have been working with a young woman on the principles outlined in this chapter. She came to me originally for weight loss, and wanted to use a non-diet approach. She has a history of an eating disorder, and at the time we first met, she felt her biggest struggle was emotional eating.

Before asking her permission to use some of her story here, I knew that she would be hesitant because in some respects, she still defines success in terms of weight loss. I don't. I feel she has been wildly successful, and I am so honored to share the tremendous growth I have seen in her.

Patrece grew up in a family that put a lot of emphasis on appearance and weight. As a young child, she was encouraged to eat less and move more in an attempt to make herself "more beautiful." That kind of environment fosters eating disorders and disordered eating, especially in children who aim to please, like Patrece. It was quite evident that she felt her worth was dependent on her weight, which led to conflicted feelings. On one hand, she wanted to lose weight because she felt her physical health would improve without extra weight. On the other hand, she was on a mission to prove that she was lovable no matter her size—a way to prove her parents and siblings wrong.

Patrece was triggered by nutrition information when we first started working together. In other words, she used it as a weapon rather than a tool. She was still prone to extremes, bouncing between rigidity and chaos. Based on her previous traumatic experiences, she was worried about what others thought and was defensive about her weight. She lacked trust and confidence in her ability to take care of herself and was externally motivated with food choices.

It was a daily process, with weekly or bimonthly sessions, but there were noticeable changes as we worked to reframe her thoughts about herself and her weight. There were two key tools used to help her establish more balanced thoughts and behaviors: self-compassion and gratitude. The first step to the extremes of rigidity or chaos is judgment. The first step back to balance is compassion. Patrece started to understand that the critical voice in her head that she thought was keeping her safe was actually making her miserable. Being patient and compassionate with herself while working through painful memories that produced faulty beliefs was her biggest asset. (I should also mention that Patrece herself is a therapist and was in therapy at this time.) Avoiding placing judgment on herself or on food allowed her to have a more balanced thought process and therefore, more balanced behaviors. She allowed herself and food to just be. "Giving up" on a diet or the diet mentality wasn't giving up at all. She was letting go of beliefs and ideas that limited her ability to be who she really was. The pendulum still swung to extremes as we worked, but Patrece was determined and dedicated. With her eye on balance, it swung less widely each time. She began to see that she could make decisions that were in her best interest, rather than base those decisions on fear, anxiety, deprivation, or restriction.

Gratitude also played a key role. Patrece started to reframe the way she thought about food. Instead of fearing it, avoiding it, calling it names, or abusing it, she started to look at food as something that nourished and fueled her body and enabled her to live a full life. She started to notice how food made her *feel*, not how it made her look. I could tell when gratitude started to take effect, and I remember vividly the day she asked for nutrition information. She was ready to use it as a tool rather than a weapon and was sincerely curious about how she could respond to her needs in a healthful way.

I don't believe if there is a point when you "arrive." I would say that being more mindful and intentional with food while practicing self-compassion and gratitude will always be a conscious choice. However, I actually feel that will be to your benefit. If making peace with food is your goal, it may take some time to rewire your subconscious judgments or learned reactions. The good news is you will have lots of opportunities to practice, and practice makes progress. I have seen self-compassion and gratitude do what nothing else could. The way you look at the problem has the power to actually change the problem itself. While this solution may sound simple, as you practice self-compassion and gratitude, I am sure you will find greater happiness and peace—results you can't argue with.

Just recently, Patrece and I made a list of what improvements she has seen. You have an idea of where she started, and this was her list of how she is feeling currently:

- feels more flow, flexibility, and balance with food, while experiencing less rigidity and frustration

- has the self-awareness to notice when she moves to extreme thoughts and behaviors and is able to respond in a more balanced way

- finds exercise that feels good and rejuvenating rather than tortuous or draining

- has less frequent headaches

- cooks at home more often; uses leftovers

- eats more satisfying breakfasts; starts self-care early in the day and is noticing a positive benefit

- is making a connection between how food makes her feel

- feels more confident in her ability to respond to what her body is truly hungry for

- uses internal motivation to drive food choices more often rather than the external motivation of manipulating food and weight

- is enjoying fruit for snacks

- sleeps improvement

- has better-quality relationships (including herself—not a coincidence!)

- is more comfortable in her own skin

- has found spiritual growth

She has expressed wanting to continue work in these and other areas. She also has her bad days when she feels discouraged, just like the rest of us. They are less frequent than before, and she can use them as an opportunity to learn and grow. My greatest hope for her is that she realizes that she is worthy of love and acceptance right now. I hope she knows this life is messy and confusing and complicated at times and that it's okay to feel overwhelmed, discouraged, and sad, but it's not okay to give up on herself. The daily practice of self-care will allow her to set and achieve realistic and truly worthwhile goals.

As you move forward, be sure to keep a big-picture approach to food. What I hope you glean from this chapter includes the following important ideas:

- Shift your mind-set from dieting and weight to self-acceptance, self-love, and self-care.

- Create a flexible structure of well-balanced meals, based on the plate method, every three to five hours using snacks based on your hunger levels. This structure is meant to be flexible, so while the plate method provides guidance, it can balance out from meal to meal and day to day to average an overall balanced approach.

- A wise place to start is to add rather than subtract. By just adding more fruits and vegetables to your meals and snacks, you will be increasing the overall nutrient density. Start adding the good to your life: food, sleep, rest, physical activity, creativity, positive thinking, and love. Focus on the good and what makes you truly happy. The rest tends to take care of itself.

- By avoiding rigid or chaotic thinking, you will avoid rigid or chaotic behavior. Instead of no cookies or ten cookies, you can take one. Instead of no ice-cream or eating the container of ice-cream, you can have a serving of ice cream after a well-balanced dinner if you would find it satisfying. You will be able to say no to foods not out of fear but out of confidence that you are making the right decision for you. You are able to say yes to foods not out of deprivation but out of confidence that you can trust your body to tell you when to stop.

- Allow yourself time to enjoy your food and let it nourish you as you slow down with meals. Turn your attention to your own innate body wisdom as you drown out the external nutrition noise around you.

- Consider the impact our relationships, emotions, and moods have on eating; remember, we are emotional beings. Utilize your emotions to care for yourself and others rather than allow negative emotions to control how you treat yourself and others.

I hope this chapter has inspired you to change the way you think about yourself and food. You have the power to create a new reality for yourself that is free of rigid or chaotic thoughts and behaviors around food. You can make the choice to take your power back and to be free of whatever hold food has on you. The way you think about food is creating your reality around it. While I realize I am taking many liberties in saying this (and please know that I understand some disease states would be an exception), I wholeheartedly believe that you choose how food affects you. The body can't lie! Believing that food will hurt you, make you sick, cause weight gain, or any other fear you have will be communicated to your body. If you see food as a potential irritant, your body will likely protect you from it. Your immune system will attack it, your digestive tract will reject it, and if you have had periods of restriction, it may want to store it to ensure adequate fuel when hunger is denied. As I stated at the beginning of this chapter, we all know what to eat. In fact, most of us are getting inundated with nutrition information constantly, villainizing a new food each time, leading us to question what there is left to eat. The best way to move forward in productive change is to get back to nutrition basics (increase nutrient density), set a flexible structure to normalize eating behaviors, and cultivate self-acceptance, self-love and self-trust. Start looking at why you eat, and be motivated out of love, not fear.

I can personally vouch for the principles I have outlined in this chapter. I attest to the power of self-acceptance and the freedom that comes with it. As I improved my relationship with myself, all of my other relationships improved exponentially, including my relationship with food. Food was (and is) my teacher, and it taught me to slow down, let love in, and find pleasure, joy, and peace by living intentionally and mindfully in the present. It is my deepest hope that you will find the same.

I often imagine a world where acceptance and love are more common than comparison and judgment. What I have realized is that it starts with us accepting and loving ourselves. "Water your own grass," as I often tell my kids. When we engage in self-care physically, emotionally, and mentally, we feel confidence and trust in our ability to make decisions in our best interest. We then will find that we trust and respect others to do the same for them. This sense of compassion and understanding for others rather than making assumptions and being divisive can literally change the world. In my little corner of the nutrition world, I hope I have changed the way you see yourself and food. I hope I have inspired you to be honest about where you are and have given you tools to meet your overall health and wellness goals.

NOTES

1. Virginia Woolf, *A Room of One's Own* (New York: Harcourt, Brace & World, 1957), 18.

2. Marci Evans, "Self-Acceptance," accessed October 12, 2013, http://marcird.com/_blog/blog/post/Self-Acceptance_The_New_Year/.

3. Linda Bacon, "Health at Every Size: The Surprising Truth About Your Weight," accessed January 26, 2015, http://www.lindabacon.org/haesbook/.

4. Ibid.

5. Linda Bacon, "The HAES Manifesto," accessed January 26, 2015, http://lindabacon.org/HAESbook/pdf_files/HAES_Manifesto.pdf.

6. Ibid.

7. Ibid.

8. "Expert Panel Recommends New Sleep Durations," *Science Daily*, accessed February 17, 2015, http://www.sciencedaily.com/releases/2015/02/150202123716.htm.

9. "ACSM Issues New Recommendations on Quantity and Quality of Exercise," *American College of Sport's Medicine*, accessed February 17, 2015, http://www.acsm.org/about-acsm/media-room/news-releases/2011/08/01/acsm-issues-new-recommendations-on-quantity-and-quality-of-exercise.

10. "Exercise 'Snacks' to Control Blood Sugar," *New York Times*, accessed February 17, 2015, http://well.blogs.nytimes.com/2014/05/14/exercise-snacks-to-control-blood-sugar/.

11. "Exercise and Immunity," *National Institutes of Health Medline Plus*, accessed February 17, 2015, http://www.nlm.nih.gov/medlineplus/ency/article/007165.htm.

12. "Statistics on Dieting and Eating Disorders," *Montenido Eating Disorder Treatment Facility*, accessed February 3, 2015, http://www.montenido.com/pdf/montenido_statistics.pdf.

13. Ibid.

14. *Narcotics Anonymous*, 1981, 11.

15. Kelly Strohacker, Katie C. Carpenter, and Brian K. McFarlin, "Consequences of Weight Cycling: An Increase in Disease Risk?" *International Journal of Exercise Science*, no. 2 (2009): 191–201.

16. K. D. Brownell and J. Rodin, "Medical, Metabolic and Psychological Effects of Weight Cycling," *Archives of Internal Medicine*, no. 154 (1994): 1325–30.

17. Strohacker, Carpenter, and McFarlin. "Consequences of Weight Cycling."

18. Daniel J. Siegel, *The Mindful Therapist* (New York: W. W. Norton & Company, 2010).

19. Barbara Rolls, *The Ultimate Volumetrics Diet* (New York: Harper Collins, 2012).

20. Jeff Novick, "A Common Sense Approach to Sound Nutrition," accessed October 12, 2013, http://www.jeffnovick.com/RD/Articles/Entries/2012/5/20_A_Common_Sense_Approach_To_Sound_Nutrition.html.

21. Rolls, *The Ultimate Volumetrics Diet*.

22. Ibid.

23. Novick, "A Common Sense Approach to Sound Nutrition."

24. Philip J. Tuso, H. Ismail, Benjamin P. Ha, and Carole Bartolotto, "Nutritional Update for Physicians: Plant-Based Diets," *The Permanente Journal*, no. 17 (2013): 61–6.

25. "Steve Jobs Always Dressed Exactly the Same. Here's Who Else Does," *Forbes*, accessed February 18, 2015, http://www.forbes.com/sites/jacquelynsmith/2012/10/05/steve-jobs-always-dressed-exactly-the-same-heres-who-else-does/.

26. Evelien van de Veer, Erica van Herpen, and Hans C. M. van Trijp, "How Do I Look? Focusing Attention on the outside body reduces responsiveness to internal signals in food intake," *Journal of Experimental Social Psychology*, no. 56 (2015): 207–13.

27. Brené Brown, *The Gifts of Imperfection* (Center City: Hazelden, 2010).

8 FITNESS FROM THE INSIDE OUT

BY KEVIN WESTON BS, ACSM EP-C

"I'VE MISSED MORE THAN NINE THOUSAND SHOTS IN MY CAREER. I'VE LOST ALMOST THREE HUNDRED GAMES. TWENTY-SIX TIMES, I'VE BEEN TRUSTED TO TAKE THE GAME WINNING SHOT AND MISSED. I'VE FAILED OVER AND OVER AND OVER AGAIN IN MY LIFE. AND THAT IS WHY I SUCCEED."[1]
—MICHAEL JORDAN

KEVIN WESTON *received his degree in exercise science from Brigham Young University and is a certified exercise physiologist from the American College of Sports Medicine and has earned certifications from the National Academy of Sports Medicine and the Cooper Institute in Dallas, Texas. He has worked professionally in the fitness industry since 2004 and is currently an exercise physiologist for the Live Well Center located at Dixie Regional Medical Center. He is pursuing a graduate degree in Applied Exercise Science from Concordia University Chicago. Kevin has written numerous articles and has appeared on multiple television spots to share his passion for exercise and human movement. Kevin and his family reside in St. George, Utah. For more information about Kevin, visit CustomFitWorkouts.com.*

Editor's note: Kevin Weston is a personal trainer and owner of Custom Fit Workouts which, as the name suggests, customizes fitness programs for a variety of client needs. I have learned that much of his philosophy stems from the same principles we promote through WholeFIT. He often tells me that mind, heart, and relationships are almost more important to your fitness goals than your actual workout. I believe the same. As we focus on what we eat and how we engage in activity combined with tapping into the power of our minds, hearts, and relationships, we will more likely reach the type of life we want to live.

INTRODUCTION

There I was, looking out the window of my west side Chicago apartment, wondering what was off with me. It was not a serious situation, but I definitely wasn't myself, and I couldn't pinpoint why I felt so sluggish, fatigued, and physically drained. I was nineteen and working as a volunteer missionary. I was originally from a small Idaho town, and even though I enjoyed my work and my new city surroundings, something was not quite right. Spiritually, mentally, and emotionally I knew I was exactly where I needed to be at that particular point in my life. However, none of that really mattered if my physical body seemed always to be running on fumes.

Over the coming weeks, I analyzed my diminished physical state, reflecting back on my childhood days. As a kid and throughout high school, I was always active and moving. I loved playing basketball, running, and doing anything outside with my friends. Active in high school sports, I was required to participate in strength conditioning classes. Although I was a typical scrawny teen who was self-conscious and loathed lifting weights, I always felt better about myself after exercise. Could exercise help improve my current physical well-being? The concept of expending energy through structured exercise to increase overall energy for the rest of the day seemed counterintuitive and misguided. How could exercise help me feel less fatigued? It made zero sense, yet I could not argue with my previous outcomes.

So one day in March 2002, I decided to give thirty minutes of daily exercise a shot. Because the mission schedule required me to wake up at 6:30 a.m., I would need to crawl out of bed by at least 6:00 a.m. if I wanted to add exercise to my already busy routine. This was going to be a sacrifice. In addition to this, I could only do exercises that could be performed inside our small apartment. Luckily there were a few random dumbbells in the apartment and a pull-up bar in one of the doorways. Starting at the crack of dawn, about four to five times a week, I went to work. I did push-ups, pull-ups, sit-ups, squats—basically anything that I could remember from my high school weight lifting class. Since we lived on the second floor, I would jump rope on the front porch to elevate my heart rate. In the beginning, the strange looks from neighbors and people walking by made me feel self-conscious, but that shyness soon evolved, as I recognized that this was a good opportunity to get acquainted with my neighbors, and I started to greet people as they passed.

Over the following months, I slowly started to notice minor changes— partly in terms of body weight but mostly in how I felt. I had more energy, had more drive, and was in a better mood. Overall I was becoming a happier person. Of course my strength and endurance improved along the way, but in my eyes, these were just a bonus. This personal experience made me think there was more to this exercise thing than just trying to get back in shape. It influenced me to make exercise and movement an important part of my personal lifestyle. It also drove me to study fitness as a career once I returned home. Daily exercise is one of many habits that, over time, has helped me become who I am today. It is a vital component of my overall health and wellness.

Now I know what you're probably thinking, but I'm not another fitness zealot who's going to guilt you into working out because you'll die prematurely if you don't. You see, when the topic of exercise is brought up in a public setting, there are typically two reactions: Some will roll their eyes, become uncomfortable, and slink away in an effort to skip the pep talk altogether. But many others have a sincere desire to inquire about health information that may help them to make life-changing decisions.

In an age where anyone can get information about any subject within seconds at the touch of a button, most people do not have the slightest clue where to start. There are so many options, they are overwhelming. If you don't believe me, type "how to lose body fat" into an Internet search, and you will receive over thirty-one million results. Thirty-one million! All different links, and much of it conflicting ideas and marketing propaganda. Is there any wonder why people's eyes glaze over when the topic of fitness and exercise is introduced? People have been feed ten pounds of bogus claims for every one pound of truth, and most don't know whom to trust anymore. Why else would anyone in their right mind buy shake weights, electronic ab belts, and diet pills? Most of us are so anxious to find the easy path to good health and a fit physique that we are always looking for that magic bullet that is as real as unicorns migrating south for the winter. Too many have lost hope that a decent quality life of will ever be realized within their lifetime.

As a fitness professional who has worked with hundreds of people of various shapes, goals, and learning styles, I have witnessed firsthand the struggles and triumphs of clients striving to improve their physical health. Two questions that I hear most frequently during the first consultation with a potential client include the following:

- "I know I need to exercise to lose weight, but I can't stay motivated. How do I change that?"

- "How long will it take to reach my goal(s)?"

The common denominator with both questions is a mind-set that exercise is purely a means to an end. If you start to exercise, good things will happen (weight loss), and preferably the sooner your goal is reached, the better so you can get back to normal life.

Unfortunately, this type of attitude toward fitness and physical activity can set you up for failure before you even start. If fitness is perceived as just another obligation that you check off from the daily to-do list, it will likely be a continual source of guilt and frustration. My goal is to help you understand how critical regular exercise is to improving *every* aspect of your life—physical, emotional, mental, and more.

The benefits of exercise are so well-documented that I think most of us know we *should* include regular exercise in our routine. In addition to the many physical benefits, exercise has also been associated with lower risk of mental illness.[3] But as I have worked and spoken with clients who drop out of regular exercise shortly after starting, there seems to be a lack of purpose or a real understanding for "why I exercise." This critical concept is often overlooked, missed, or ignored. If a client's only reason for going to the gym, on a walk, or for a bike ride is to solely to fit back into their skinny jeans before their twenty-year high school reunion in six weeks, the likelihood of sticking with it beyond *the event* is greatly in doubt.

This concept of focusing on your *why* instead of just the *result* you want (losing twenty pounds, for example) will not diminish your ultimate outcome. Instead, it will allow you to instill habits that become ingrained into your everyday behavior, not just out-of-the-ordinary activities you are doing until you reach your goal. The desired outcomes you seek can happen indirectly as you do the little things, accumulated over a period of time, day in and day out.

At the start of each new calendar year, millions of people make New Year's resolutions to lose weight, defining success solely based on if they lose weight or not in the first few months or so. Research suggests that 50 percent of those who start exercising will stop within the first six months.[4] I was actually surprised the percentage wasn't higher. You've probably witnessed this yourself; your local gym is a zoo in January and a ghost town in June. There are many reasons, but I would like to think that one of the most common reasons people give up on exercise is that changing your body composition (losing weight, gaining muscle, and so on) is really hard, and it takes more time and commitment than most people realize. So if you're only motivated by how quickly the number on the bathroom scale drops, brace yourself for a lesson in human physiology, especially if you want to maintain those results long term. Again, if you want to succeed at achieving better health, and you want this lifestyle change to be permanent, you'll need to focus on changes you are willing to implement that are sustainable. In other words, are you motivated enough that you could keep this up for years instead of weeks? If not, it's time to put the horse in front of the cart, not the other way around.

WHAT MOTIVATES PEOPLE TO EXERCISE?

The science of exercise is evolving like any other field of study. One prominent study by Trost and colleagues reviewed previous participation and exercise adherence studies and designated five categories that influence exercise motivation: (1) demographic and biological factors, (2) psychological, cognitive and emotional factors, (3) behavioral attributes and skills, (4) social and cultural influences, and (5) physical environment and/or physical activity characteristics.[5] In essence, people are motivated for different reasons and what drives one individual to be active may not influence another.

I believe only you can truly discover your exercise "why," and there will definitely be some trial and error along the way. Maybe you want to be physically able to play with your grandchildren or have the stamina to travel the world or just feel better overall. There are countless reasons for why people adhere to long-term daily activity. A key to your lifelong fitness success is a willingness to accept and embrace the challenges you will surely face as you find out what truly moves you to be active every day.

YOUR GOALS AND YOUR "WHY" STATEMENTS SHOULD BE DIFFERENT

On the surface, you may assume that goals and "why I exercise" purposes are basically the same thing, right? Not exactly, and here's why: Over time, goals change, but the fundamental reason or "why" a lifelong exerciser is active every day is unchanging. If a person's primary motivation for structured exercise is a driven desire to feel better, have more energy, or have increased independence, then individual goals become checkpoints on the road rather than the finish line. For example, a fifty-eight-year-old female can say her "why" is to be physically capable to care for her aging parents and go hiking with her grandchildren. She also has a goal to lose twenty pounds in three months. Let's say she loses eight pounds. Is she a failure? Should she not have started in the first place? Was all her walking, swimming, and dumbbell curling done in vain? Will someone else need to take care of her parents or hike with her grandkids because she is only 8 pounds lighter? Of course not! When one has a well-thought and truly ingrained "why I exercise" purpose, success is not contingent on the results of individual goals. You may fail at achieving a specific goal, without failing your "why." You can adjust, tweak, or sometimes completely change your goals that will evolve over the course of your life, because overall, goals support your underlying "why."

5 TIPS TO START WITH TODAY

1. Do active things that you enjoy.

Too many times, people will perform certain types of exercise programs that they've heard will help them lose weight, gain muscle, trim this, and tone that. However, deep down inside, they really despise the program. If you hate running for example, don't start running as your primary means of exercise because that is what your friend did to reach his or her goal. Instead, find activities that you enjoy doing that may not necessarily feel like exercise. Sometimes the most unconventional approach to fitness can be the most effective. Get outside, go dancing, walk nine holes of golf, rock climb, learn martial arts—whatever you will at least tolerate will be your best bet going forward. If you're going to be consistent with exercise and in it for the long haul, start with what you like doing now. A simple way to gauge your commitment is seeing how well you maintain your activity levels during disruptions of your regular schedule. Examples of this include vacations or having visitors at your home for an extended period of time. If you like an activity well enough, you'll look for excuses to participate rather than looking for excuses to skip out on a specific activity. Spend a few months (maybe even a year if necessary) learning to be consistent with activities you truly enjoy before setting goals that require activities that are not necessarily your favorites.

2. Strive for thirty minutes a day.

The American College of Sports Medicine recommends that adults get one hundred and fifty minutes a week (five days per week, thirty minutes per day) of moderate intense exercise for chronic disease prevention and weight management.[6] Although weight loss outcomes may require more time than thirty minutes, the first step is to start with activities you know you can make habitual. The ACSM also points out that your daily thirty minutes of activity does not have to be done consecutively. It can be broken up into two or three smaller ten-to-fifteen minute segments. You have to start somewhere. The key is to find an approach that works for you that you can maintain long term.

3. Break up screen time.

As a nation, we are literally sitting ourselves to death.[7] The human body is designed to move, not be constantly plopped in front of a computer, TV, phone, tablet, or anything with a screen. It is recommended to reduce prolonged sedentary behavior to no more than sixty minutes at a time and break it up with bouts of any intensity activity.[8] Even if you are exercising thirty minutes a day, the benefits are reduced if you are largely sedentary the other fifteen-and-a-half hours of the day. This phenomenon is known as being an "active couch potato." Starkoff and Lenz suggest breaking up these periods of prolonged sitting with multiple short bursts of activity to improve blood pressure, waist circumference, triglycerides, and glucose metabolism.

I personally interpret this recommendation to be finding opportunities to break away from the tech world and to get up, stretch, walk, and move around multiple times throughout the day. This is encouraged at work, at home, and during leisure time.

4. Focus on sustainability.

When potential clients brag to me about extreme diets, exercise machines, or anything else that helped them to lose weight they have since gained back, I follow up with this question: "How did that work for you?" Of course I already know they were following some unsustainable protocol that they didn't have a prayer of maintaining, but it opens up dialogue regarding what is real change and what is just a quick fix. If people cannot see themselves doing something for the rest of their lives, there's a chance that what they're doing is a facade. It's not real change in the sense of becoming healthier individuals. Rather, it's just faking being healthy for a brief period of time. When considering new activities or programs, ask yourself, "Can I see myself doing this five, ten, or fifteen years down the road?" If not, you may want to look at other options.

5. Embrace the process.

I don't mean for this chapter to be a cliché "enjoy the journey" tagline for fitness. My key point is that fitness requires long-term commitment to processes that will greatly influence much more than just your physical health. Listen, if there were truly an alternative to exercise that had the same number of long- and short-term benefits, we would all be doing it. As humans, our bodies are designed to move, walk, climb, and experience all that this amazing world has to offer. Embrace the process of change from the inside out. Make the investment in yourself.

As a young nineteen-year-old teenager struggling in Chicago with my physical well-being, I discovered the emotional, intellectual, and mental benefits of exercise. I know that changing behavior can be hard, and sometimes it can be downright discouraging. Yet somewhere along the way, you realize it's truly worth the daily price you pay to be your overall best. Now is the time to make the necessary preparations to incorporate more activity in your daily routine. Let today become the beginning of a lifestyle of movement.

NOTES

1. Michael Jordan, "Failure," commercial for Nike, accessed October 23, 2015, https://www.youtube.com/watch?v=GuXZFQKKF7A.

2. Jack Dixon, as quoted in David DeFord *1000 Brilliant Achievement Quotes: Advice from the World's Wisest* (Omaha, NE: Ordinary People Can Win!, 2004), 74.

3. G. Cooney et al., "Exercise for Depression," September 13, 2013, http://www.cochrane.org/CD004366/DEPRESSN_exercise-for-depression.

4. K. Wilson and D. Brooksfield, "Effect of Goal Setting on Motivation and Adherence in a Six-week Exercise Program," *International Journal of Sport and Exercise Physiology* 7, no. 1 (2009): 89–100.

5. S. G. Trost et al, "Correlates of Adults' participation in Physical Activity: Review and Update," *Medicine & Science in Sports & Exercise* 34, no. 12 (2002).

6. "Quantity and Quality of Exercise for Developing and Maintaining Cardiorespiratory, Musculoskeletal, and Neuromotor Fitness in Apparently Healthy Adults: Guidance for Prescribing Exercise," *Medicine & Science in Sports & Exercise* 43, no. 7 (2011): 1334–59.

7. Chai Woodham, "Are You Sitting Yourself to Death?" Health.UsNews.com, May 2, 2012, http://health.usnews.com/health-news/articles/2012/05/02/are-you-sitting-yourself-to-death.

8. Brooke Starkoff and Elizabeth Lenz, "Improving Health by Breaking Up Continuous Bouts of Sedentary Behavior," *ACSM Health & Fitness Journal* 19, no. 2 (2015): 14–19.

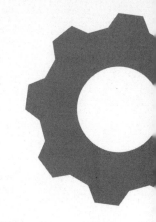

9 TAKING CONTROL OF YOUR HEALTH

BY MICHAEL ANDERSON, MD; JR MARTIN, PA;
& W. JARED DUPREE, PHD, MBA

"WHAT LIES BEHIND US AND WHAT LIES BEFORE US ARE TINY MATTERS COMPARED TO WHAT LIES WITHIN US."[1] —HENRY S. HASKINS

"THERE ARE THINGS WE CAN CONTROL, THINGS WE CAN AFFECT, AND THINGS WE CAN'T CONTROL." —DR. MICHAEL ANDERSON

MICHAEL ANDERSON, MD, *has been practicing in St. George, Utah, for more than twenty-five years, making him the senior-most orthopedic surgeon in all of Southern Utah. His special interest in hip and knee replacement surgery began early in his career while training at the University of Utah under the tutelage of some of the foremost pioneers in joint replacement surgery, including Aaron Hofmann, MD, Kent Samuelson, MD, and Harold Dunn, MD. Dr. Anderson is also the longest-serving member of the American Association of Hip and Knee Surgeons (AAHKS) in Southern Utah. He is certified by the American Board of Orthopaedic Surgery (ABOS).*

For fifteen years Dr. Anderson and his partners provided Sports Medicine coverage for Dixie State University and the local area high schools, donating time and expertise to keep the student athletes on the field and in the game. As a part of that service, knowledge and proficiency in the latest arthroscopic techniques of the knee and shoulder have been offered to the Washington County area athletes. Dr. Anderson continues to enjoy the "bread and butter" of general orthopedics, hand surgery, carpal tunnel, and trigger fingers, and the unpredictable challenge of trauma and piecing back together broken bones.

In the last year of medical school at the University of Utah, Dr. Anderson's life focus broadened when his future wife, Kelly, walked through the door. Thirty years and four boys later, they've made their home in Southern Utah. His love of the out of doors, climbing, cycling, and photography have filled the time not taken by his practice of medicine.

*His training in orthopedic surgery has given him some unique opportunities, including serving as the crew physician for an IMAX film in Antarctica documenting the 1914 travels of Ernest Shackleton (*Shackleton's Antarctic Adventure*), as well as volunteer work in third-world countries.*

JR MARTIN, PA, *received his bachelor of science in chemistry and master of science in health promotion from Brigham Young University. Later, he received a master of medical science from Midwestern University and eventually became licensed as a physician's assistant (PA). He worked at Enterprise Valley Medical Center between 2002 and 2005 and later worked for the Emergency Department at Dixie Regional Medical Center in St. George, Utah, between 2006 and 2015. He is the founder of Alive & Well, which began in 1995 and has begun to work full-time to provide individuals, families, and corporations total solutions to their health and wellness. JR has competed in various types of running, triathlon and cycling events and is a self-described family man.*

Editor's note: I first met JR Martin at an early morning breakfast at a restaurant close to the hospital where we both worked. The purpose of our meeting was a discussion about how some of the principles of WholeFIT could relate to his new initiative called Alive & Well. He explained to me how frustrated he had become with watching people come to the ER with conditions that could be prevented. Emergency Room visits can be extremely costly (at this writing, the average visit costs $1500 or more), and JR wanted to see his patients avoid that kind of expense. He also felt frustrated about the fact that if he had been able to work with and counsel with patients five years earlier (or even a single year earlier), the ER visit might have been prevented altogether. "It's not right," he said. "I didn't get into this profession to put Band-Aids on issues that go deeper than their current symptoms. I want to help people for real." JR was so passionate about his desire to truly help people with preventative health care that he quit a high-paying ER job to dedicate all of his professional time to helping individuals, families and companies access affordable health care that focuses on the long term.

Both JR and Dr. Anderson have experienced wellness on a personal level, and in the following pages, you'll learn how to duplicate their success.

JR'S STORY

It is 7:00 a.m. on May 1, 2010. I find myself shivering in a sea of swimmers. The water in Sand Hollow reservoir is a chilly sixty-two degrees. The starting cannon booms. The first full Saint George Iron Man has begun. Suddenly, I feel like I am in a blender. Swimmers make their cut past, under, and over me.

I wonder if I am having an out-of-body experience. A smile breaks out across my face as I lean forward and submerge myself. At first my mind flashes back to what brought me to this point. Within a couple of strokes my thoughts race to the cone that lies ahead. And somewhere in the middle of what lies behind and what lies before, I begin to think of what lies within me. I remember saying to myself, "I guess I am going to find out if I can really do this."

WHAT LIES BEHIND

Perhaps it was the craziness of a 2.4-mile swim, 112-mile bike ride, or 26.2-mile run that attracted me. Perhaps it was the fact that the bike course traveled right past my home. Perhaps it was a midlife crisis and an expanding gut. Perhaps it was the date. I have always been a little quirky and superstitious. (I left on a mission for the LDS Church on May 1, so that date always had special meaning to me). Whatever it was, somehow it all came together and piqued my desire. Before I could back out, I paid my entrance fee and registered for the ride of my life. Now the training would begin

Past experiences made me feel comfortable with the run. But the swim and bicycling sent shivers down my spine. I decided to start training with what scared me the most!

I was petrified of the swim. Simply put, I can't swim. I thought I would die when I had to swim the mile as a scout. It took me forever. I was literally one of the last ones out of the water in two previous triathlons. Thankfully, a friend warned me my wetsuit was on backward prior to one event. I felt like a moron.

So I started to train with the swim. Each morning, I made my way to the local pool, towel in hand. The swimming was slow and painful. Gradually, I worked my way up to a full mile. Then to two miles. One day, I slapped the water in delight when I had actually completed the entire 2.4 miles in less than the cut-off time for the event. I knew the water at Sand Hollow would be much different than the pool. But I had hope. Maybe I could do this!

Next the bike. I had no experience with road biking. I borrowed my neighbor's bike because I had none of my own. I decided to train on the course as much as possible. The day of my first attempt on the course, I nearly talked myself out of the triathlon. I distinctly remember thinking that Steve, a close friend of mine, would not want me to train or do the Iron Man. I imagined his disgust with my selfish investment of time and effort. Maybe I should quit rather than disappoint him. Then it struck me. I was cold. I was tired. It was dark. I was scared. Wait a minute, it wasn't my friend who wanted me to quit, it was me that wanted to quit. I was placing my friend as the scapegoat. The truth was Steve had no idea that I was even training. Plus, I had no idea what he really thought. The realization that I was making excuses outside of myself (for myself) was a defining moment. I actually talked out loud and began to laugh. "You don't want to quit because of Steve. You want to quit because you're cold and tired." After I began to deal with my internal struggle, training became an adventure. What would

I find out about myself today? What obstacle may present itself for me to overcome?

The hills on the bike route are appropriately named "Mini Bitch" and "The Wall." For months, I could not get up either hill without getting off my bike and walking. Sometimes I was so tired I would pull the bike off the road and lie down and sleep. Another breakthrough came when I realized my tires were inflated only half of what they should be. I felt like a Clydesdale horse who had been pulling the Budweiser Beer trailer in the sand. Once the tires were inflated, I could fly! Like magic, I was able to make it up each hill without getting off the bike. My new mantra became "Just stay on the bike."

I would run to and from work at all hours of the night. Soon enough, the event was just weeks away. At some point I made a commitment: "I won't quit." I might be pulled off the course for medical reasons or because I was simply too slow. But I decided that nothing else would stop me.

WHAT LIES AHEAD

As I made my way from cone to cone in the water, I was sweetly surprised. I was making the cut off times! "Hey, I may actually make the swim" I thought to myself. Sure enough, I made it out of the water! I had time to spare. My adrenaline soared as I approached my bike.

I couldn't hold back the excitement as I passed other bikers with reckless abandonment. Discipline was thrown out the door out of the joy of not drowning.

Six miles into the 112-mile bike ride, disaster struck. My derailleur snapped. My bike and my hopes came to a screeching halt. Was it all over? My heart sank as other bikers whipped by me. I felt sad, lonely, stranded, and stuck. I was told there was help at the bottom of the hill. Out of desperation, I coasted back down the mile-long hill I had just climbed as a field of bikers all heading the proper direction passed me. Finally, I was told that my bike could be fixed but just to one gear. I was asked what gear I wanted it set at. I responded "something in the middle." Then the moment of truth came.

I knew what was behind me (all the training, all the time, all the pain); I knew what was ahead of me (106 miles, Mini Bitch, The Wall) and a marathon to run. But both of those things were actually tiny things compared to what was within me—a commitment to not quit. So off I went.

All I really had was my commitment. I had no idea if I could make it. Amazingly, however, it didn't seem to matter. All that mattered was honoring what was in me.

Myriad events and circumstances ensued over the course of the next sixteen hours and five minutes. Ultimately, I crossed the line at 11:06 p.m. into the arms of my beautiful wife. I actually finished the race.

So why do I tell you this story? It is certainly not because I am a great athlete or unusual. It is precisely because I am an average athlete and a very usual kind of guy.

Each of us, regardless of our circumstances, will encounter experiences in life that pose obstacles. Sometimes the obstacles will be things we can change, sometimes not. There are circumstances we can alter and circumstances we can't. As James Allen states in his book *As a Man Thinketh*, "circumstance reveals a man to himself."[2]

We may not be able to control if and when our bicycle derailleur snaps. But we can control how we react if and when the things we can't control happen.

The key to our success is to commit to the things we can control. The things we can control are never outside of ourselves. The things we can control are within us. Commit to keep going. Commit to keep trying. Commit to keep learning.

The commitment to discover and stay true to what lies within us prepares us for the greatest ride of our lives!

WHAT CAN WE CONTROL?

Over the course of nearly thirty years of practicing orthopedic surgery, I have learned many lessons from my patients. I've tried to look for threads of consistency in my experiences with patients to piece together things that I may learn from or share with others for their benefit.

Here's one example: When someone says, "Here, hold my beer, watch this!" something bad is usually about to occur. If a person of limited judgment—the young, the inebriated, or the impaired—takes the controls of a motorized recreational vehicle, I will often acquire a new patient.

There's another truth I like to share with my patients, which has come from my experience watching other people make choices. Here's what I've learned:

- Control the things you can control.

- Influence the things you can influence.

- Understand there are things you cannot control.

Many patients could save themselves money and multiple trips to the doctor, avoid a lot of grief, and live more enjoyable lives if they just controlled the things they can control. Let me explain further by identifying two common problems that seem to travel in tandem to my office each clinic day. The first is *inactivity*. Its sibling is *obesity*. Both of these fall into the category of *things we can control* or at the very least influence, and for those who fail to control these twin demons, the results are devastating and usually inescapable.

INACTIVITY

The facts: Inactivity is linked directly to obesity, diabetes, coronary artery disease, breast cancer, depression, and a number of other common illnesses. If physical inactivity rates were to go down by 20 percent, we could save well over 1 million lives in one year. Imagine the incalculable health benefits for the millions of others whose lives would be prolonged by such a significant change for good. Recent Harvard studies on inactivity documented that one-third of adults and close to 80 percent of adolescents worldwide are at increased risk of disease as result of physical inactivity. Further, 1.5 billion adults worldwide face a 20 to 30 percent increased risk of heart disease, diabetes, and other health-related problems. Numerous studies indicate that inactivity tends to rise with age and is more common with women than men.

Early in my career, I had the opportunity to work at the Veterans Hospital in Salt Lake City. I remember distinctly one particular patient, a seventy-four-year-old right-handed retiree, who was evaluated for sore shoulder. I inquired, "So how did you hurt your shoulder?"

He quickly responded, "I was carrying a bucket of cement and something just tore."

He winced with a muscle spasm, and I couldn't help but ask, "You are seventy-four years old. What are you doing carrying a bucket of cement?"

To that he responded, "My dad and I are building a garage." Assuming his father was well into his nineties and also very active has served as a testament to me of the importance of a commitment to regular, vigorous activity.

OBESITY

Associated with inactivity but a separate problem is that of obesity.

Control Your Weight

Looking to get to or stay at a healthy weight? Both diet and physical activity play a critical role in controlling your weight. You gain weight when the calories you burn, including those burned during physical activity, are less than the calories you eat or drink. When it comes to weight management, people vary greatly in how much physical activity they need. You may need to be more active than others to achieve or maintain a healthy weight. Activity alone does not accomplish the goal of improved or ideal body weight. Dietary changes have to be paired with activity or the process will not work.

Considering the fact that obesity may be the greatest epidemic in the history of planet earth, not enough of us are doing something about it. Numerous studies document that obesity is on the rise in the world, and in America it is increasing even faster. Obesity is defined as having a BMI (body mass index) greater than thirty. The broad effects of obesity touch almost every aspect of a person's health. The causes are discussed throughout this book. They are multifactorial and include a heavy genetic component, family history, metabolic and disease-related causes, as well as a strong emotional and psychological component.

Obesity has been shown to be highly correlated with various diseases, including type 2 diabetes, breast cancer, heart disease, obstructive sleep apnea, and osteoarthritis. It is a leading preventable cause of death worldwide, and sadly the rates of obesity are skyrocketing. At the present time 60 percent of the US population is judged overweight, 30 percent are obese, and a significant portion of those fall in the category of morbidly obese. Sadly it wasn't until 2013 that the American Medical Association finally classified obesity as a disease. You have heard this weight loss advice mentioned by other contributors to this book. I will mention it yet again because it is so important.

1. *To maintain your weight:* Work your way up to 150 minutes of moderate-intensity aerobic activity, 75 minutes of vigorous-intensity aerobic activity, or an equivalent mix of the two each week. Strong scientific evidence shows that physical activity can help you maintain your weight over time. However, the exact amount of physical activity needed to do this is not clear because it varies greatly from person to person. It's possible that you may need to do more than the equivalent of 150 minutes of moderate-intensity activity a week to maintain your weight.

2. *To lose weight and keep it off:* You will need a high amount of physical activity unless you also adjust your diet and reduce the amount of calories you're eating and drinking. The right combination of weekly activity and dietary changes are essential. Getting to and staying at a healthy weight requires both regular physical activity and a healthy eating plan. The CDC has some great tools and information about nutrition, physical activity, and weight loss. Emily has given

some great recommendations on nutrition in chapter 7, and the recommendations for fitness from chapter 8 will also be helpful if you haven't read, or would like to review this information.

WHY SHOULD WE ADDRESS INACTIVITY & OBESITY?

Reduce Your Risk of Cardiovascular Disease

Heart disease and stroke are two of the leading causes of death in the United States. But following the guidelines and getting at least 150 minutes a week (2 hours and 30 minutes) of moderate-intensity aerobic activity can put you at a lower risk for these diseases. You can reduce your risk even further with more physical activity. Regular physical activity can also lower your blood pressure and improve your cholesterol levels.

Reduce Your Risk of Type 2 Diabetes and Metabolic Syndrome

Regular physical activity can reduce your risk of developing type 2 diabetes and metabolic syndrome. Metabolic syndrome is a condition in which you have some combination of too much fat around the waist, high blood pressure, low HDL cholesterol, high triglycerides, or high blood sugar. Research shows that lower rates of these conditions are seen with 120 to 150 minutes (2 hours to 2 hours and 30 minutes) a week of at least moderate-intensity aerobic activity. And the more physical activity you do, the lower your risk will be. Already have type 2 diabetes? Regular physical activity can help control your blood glucose levels as well.

Reduce Your Risk of Some Cancers

Research shows that physically active people have a lower risk of colon cancer, and physically active women have a lower risk of breast cancer. Although the research is not yet final, some findings suggest that you can also reduce your risk of endometrial and lung cancer by being physically active. If you are a cancer survivor, research shows that getting regular physical activity not only helps give you a better quality of life but also improves your physical fitness.

Strengthen Your Bones and Muscles

As you age, it's important to protect your bones, joints, and muscles. Not only do they support your body and help you move, but keeping bones, joints, and muscles healthy can help ensure that you're able to do your daily activities and be physically active. Research shows that doing aerobic, muscle-strengthening and bone-strengthening physical activity of at least a moderately intense level can slow the loss of bone density that comes with age.

Hip fracture is a serious health condition that can have life-changing negative effects, especially if you're an older adult. But research shows that people who do 120 to 300 minutes of at least moderate-intensity aerobic activity each week have a lower risk of hip fracture.

Regular physical activity helps with arthritis and other conditions affecting the joints. If you have arthritis, research shows that doing 130 to 150 (2 hours and 10 minutes to 2 hours and 30 minutes) a week of moderate-intensity, low-impact aerobic activity can not only improve your ability to manage pain and do everyday tasks, but it can also make your quality of life better.

Build strong, healthy muscles. Muscle-strengthening activities can help you increase or maintain your muscle mass and strength. Slowly increasing the amount of weight and number of repetitions you do will give you even more benefits, no matter your age.

Improve Your Mental Health and Mood

Regular physical activity can help keep your thinking, learning, and judgment skills sharp as you age. It can also reduce your risk of depression and may help you sleep better. Research has shown that doing aerobic or a mix of aerobic and muscle-strengthening activities three to five times a week for thirty to sixty minutes can give you these mental health benefits. Some scientific evidence has also shown that even lower levels of physical activity can be beneficial.

Improve Your Ability to Do Daily Activities and Prevent Falls

I've found that middle-aged and older individuals who ride bicycles, (not a stationary bike) seem to have improved balance and agility, hence, fewer falls. Another side benefit is that riding a bike is a very efficient method for burning calories without the wear and tear on weight-bearing joints. Risks with cycling are that you can fall off the bike or get hit by a car or another cyclists, leading to serious injury. Before engaging in cycling, it is important that you are given approval by your primary care physician.

A functional limitation as you age is a loss of the ability to do everyday activities such as climbing stairs, grocery shopping, or playing with your grandchildren. Committing to a course of regular activity slows this inevitable process of functional limitations.

Are you an older adult who is at risk for falls? Research shows that doing balance and muscle-strengthening activities each week along with moderate-intensity aerobic activity, like brisk walking, can help reduce your risk of falling. Again cycling, if you have adequate balance, may be a tool for you to maintain your independence.

Increase Your Chances of Living Longer

Science shows that physical activity can reduce your risk of dying early from the leading causes of death, like heart disease and some cancers. Only a few life-style choices have as large an impact on your health as physical activity. People who are physically active for about seven hours a week have a 40 percent lower risk of dying early than those who are active for less than thirty minutes a week. You don't have to do high amounts of activity or vigorous-intensity activity to reduce your risk of premature death. You can put yourself at lower risk of dying early by doing at least 150 minutes a week of moderate-intensity aerobic activity.

TAKE CONTROL OF WHAT YOU CAN

The two important health factors of obesity and inactivity usually fall into the category of either, "I can control them" or at the very least, "I can influence them." Both obesity and inactivity are not stand-alone entities but rather fit comfortably within the definition of a syndrome, namely: "A group of signs and symptoms that occur together to characterize a particular abnormality." As mentioned above, inactivity and obesity have numerous problems, either directly or indirectly related to them.

A frustration I've seen as a practitioner of medicine is when people don't get the connection between the things they can control or influence and the ones they can't. For example, one day in clinic an overweight patient was being evaluated for his knees and hips as well as general aches and pains. He patted his moist forehead with a napkin as he expressed puzzlement over his condition. "I don't understand where this weight comes from. I'm so active; every weekend I'm out on my four-wheeler, and yet I still gain weight. I just don't understand." He followed that with a wry smile and said, "I guess for my age I'm doing okay." He was four years younger than me. This patient has given up his agency. He was making choice not to control or influence the things he could.

To complete the discussion, some words need to be said concerning those things that we cannot control. For example, if a drunk driver happens to hit you or a family member, there's not much you can do about that. I refer to that as "when lightning strikes." Some things are beyond your control. We shouldn't expend our energy worrying about things we cannot control. Certain health conditions just happen for any one of a number of reasons. No point in worrying about them.

Now is the time to take control of those things in your life that you can control and enjoy the challenge of trying to influence the other factors that will make life more fun and fulfilling and maybe even prolong it.

 ACTION ITEMS

Health-care providers are trained to help people stay well, and while there is still much to learn, a lot of what we know about staying healthy isn't rocket science. There are no magic pills or quick fixes. Instead, each of us has to have the desire to take control of our health and live in a way that taps into the natural resources and strengths our bodies already provide. There is not much we can do about those areas of life outside of our control, but we offer some final suggestions that are in your control:

1. **Decide now to take control of your health.** There are many excuses, road-blocks, and challenges to making a change. As we attempt to get out of our comfort zone and make a lifestyle change, thoughts will come to our minds that tell us to stop. Emotions will rise that will tempt us to quit. Pain will surface that will ask for rest. Although it may take time, make a decision to push through. You *can* be in control.

2. **Take baby steps.** Despite of being afraid and unsure of his ability to learn to swim, JR started by taking a towel and getting himself to the pool. He started slow and exerted a little more effort each time until he reached a goal he originally thought was unattainable. It's okay to start slow; it's more important that you get on the path and keep walking that journey.

3. **Prioritize 150 minutes or more a week of activity.** Thirty minutes of activity, five days a week is doable for almost any of us. Do you honestly have any excuse for *not* finding that much time for self care? It seems almost too simple that these few minutes of prevention and protection could offer so many health benefits, yet they do! Implementing this one small course correction may save your life. It will likely help you be happier as well!

4. **Remember that healthy weight is about healthy living.** We aren't really into dieting or fad programs, but we do know our weight can impact our health. We want to be clear that we aren't suggesting a certain body type or set of measurements as it relates to body image. Rather, we are suggesting that engaging in activity and healthy eating will naturally help you reach the weight that is right for you.

FINAL THOUGHTS

We only have one life to live. There are ups and downs in this journey we call life. Things will happen. Pain, disappointment, accidents, bad luck—these will come. Happiness, balance, and peace can come as well. We believe that letting go of those areas out of our control and embracing what has been given to us that is in our control can help. We hope you can take hold of the courage inside of you and do the little things that matter most. In the end, our health allows us to enjoy what is most important in life—our families, serving others, and engaging in what we love.

NOTES

1. Henry S. Haskins, *Meditations in Wall Street* (New York: William Morrow & Company, 1940).

2. J. Allen, *As a Man Thinketh* (New York: Thomas Y. Crowell Company, 1913).

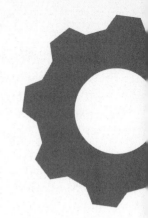

10 LIVING WELL WITH CHRONIC ILLNESS

BY JENNIFER HARSH, PHD; MARK B. WHITE, PHD;
& LISA TYNDALL, PHD

"EVERYONE WHO IS BORN HOLDS DUAL CITIZENSHIP, IN THE KINGDOM OF THE WELL AND IN THE KINGDOM OF THE SICK. ALTHOUGH WE ALL PREFER TO USE ONLY THE GOOD PASSPORT, SOONER OR LATER EACH OF US IS OBLIGED, AT LEAST FOR A SPELL, TO IDENTIFY OURSELVES AS CITIZENS OF THAT OTHER PLACE."[1] —SUSAN SONTAG

Editor's note: These authors remind us that each of us will pass through sickness and disease during our lives—some of us more than others. How we live and make sense of what is given to us can make all the difference. If you or a loved one are dealing with a chronic illness, please consider this chapter as you press forward on your journey. Small and simple things at times can make all the difference.

INTRODUCTION

Jessica remembers that day as if it were yesterday. She and her husband, Karl, were sitting in Dr. Garcia's office. Fortunately she had been able to get dressed and move from the cold, sterile examination room to Dr. Garcia's office to hear the verdict. The news that she had breast cancer became an event that bisected her life into two segments: before cancer and after cancer.

Variations on this story exist for tens of thousands of individuals each year who discover they have a chronic condition for which they'll need to receive ongoing medical care. In 2012, the Centers for Disease Control estimated that about half of all adults in the United States have one or more chronic conditions (such as heart disease, stroke, cancer, obesity).[2] For some, the diagnosis is sudden and unanticipated. Others have had symptoms for years, and a recent diagnosis has finally given a name to a condition they have suffered with for some time. A chronic condition impacts every facet of a patient's life, including work, relationships with family members and friends, caring for children, finances, and a person's free time.

In our research and clinical work, we have seen individuals, couples, and families manage the physical and emotional aspects of chronic illness in different ways. Some seem consistently resilient from the onset, others struggle from crisis to crisis, and yet others emerge from a valley of challenges, stronger and seemingly refined by fire. Over time, each person and each family determines their own set of coping mechanisms. That said, there seems to be no right or wrong way to cope. Through an often hard-fought process, people can discover how to use their own unique strengths, and the strengths of their family and friends, to determine how they'd like to define, achieve, and maintain well-being. Common themes emerge when people navigate the chronic illness experience, whether it is their own or that of a loved one. The following are brief descriptions of a handful of these themes.

MAKING MEANING

When facing an illness or disability, a range of questions often emerge: Why am I the one who has diabetes, when my diet is so healthy compared to everyone else's? What does having cancer mean for who I am and how I live my life? How will my family understand that because of my multiple sclerosis (MS) I won't always be able to participate in activities that we enjoy?

These are questions that people with chronic medical difficulties may ask themselves when they're newly diagnosed or over the course of their illness. For example, when individuals with multiple sclerosis (MS) were asked why they believed they developed MS, they attributed their illness to a host of factors, including a germ or virus, stress, pollution, a family history of MS, or punishment from God for their sins. A few responded with "why *not* me?"[3] For this last group of respondents, MS was just another trial in life that could happen to anyone. Why would they be immune from challenges?

A diagnosis of a chronic illness will cause myriad questions and conflicting feelings. These feelings may arise from within the ill person, may be driven by family members and friends, or may reflect sentiments prevalent in society. Gaining an understanding of what an illness experience *means* to a person and how the illness may or may not shape that person's life can be an important first step in coping. The research generally finds that those who manage to find some kind of personal meaning in their illness experience fare better over time than those who do not engage in attempts to discover what their illness means to the way in which they now must live their life. So, what does it *mean* to *make meaning*? We would suggest that meaning making involves a few key elements: mourning, acceptance, finding benefits, and refashioning a new life.

Mourning

When diagnosed with an illness or when an individual is experiencing difficult physical symptoms, it takes time and effort to mourn the loss of a once-healthy life. For many, the mourning experience is similar to mourning the loss of a job or a relationship or experiencing the death of a loved one. The loss of your health is extremely impactful and deserves the time and attention that any other loss in life garners. Taking the time and spending the energy to grieve this loss of health can be a powerful coping tool and can set a person up for beginning to accept the set of difficulties illness can bring. Like any other part of the illness experience, mourning the loss of health can take many forms. For example, some people find comfort in sharing their feelings and experiences with loved ones, other find that quiet reflection is an important ingredient in the mourning experience, and still others find that both external discussion and internal reflection are needed in the grieving process.

Acceptance

Like grieving, acceptance looks different for each person. People can choose to accept things in stages, accept some parts of the diagnosis but not others, or quickly move to embrace this significant change in their lives. In his work with mindfulness, Kabat-Zinn described acceptance as a way to facilitate moving into the next best step. In other words, coming to terms with the facts of the diagnosis as it currently is, or as each day comes (rather than fretting uselessly about what will happen two or five or ten years from now) allows a person to be more fully present and to determine what course of action is truly the best for the immediate situation.[4] Acceptance does not mean resigning yourself to *accept* a given prognosis or set of limitations with whatever illness is being faced. But coming to terms with the illness experience, as it is each day, can help a person to discover what can be changed, take action to implement those changes, and then accept what cannot be changed.

Finding Benefits

Can there really be benefits to having a chronic illness? We think so, and we have seen many people with various types of illness who have found real benefits in their lives. Many discover that having a chronic illness helps them to gain perspective, which can in turn increase overall perceived well-being. Perspective allows you to let go of a tendency to be distressed over the "little" things like not receiving a raise at work or being cut off in traffic, because another concern (maintaining physical health) looms larger. Likewise, a sense of purpose may begin to emerge that is different than a person's prechronic illness ideas about their purpose in life. Many people find a community of others with similar illnesses. They may fundraise, participate in events, and speak publically about their own illness experience. There has also been a significant body of research on posttraumatic growth, the notion that growth and change can happen as a result of struggling with a traumatic event. As we face these crises, we may discover new ways to live our life, feel increased appreciation for life and close relationships, and come to the realization that we are stronger than we initially thought we were.[5]

Refashioning a New Life

Refashioning a new life, or creating a new normal, can be quite challenging. The aforementioned aspects of coping, mourning, acceptance, and finding benefits all play instrumental roles. Ultimately, it involves living a full and complete postdiagnosis life: priorities have shifted, relationships have deepened, losses have been mourned, health has been redefined, and new hobbies and recreational activities are in place.

KNOWLEDGE ABOUT ILLNESS

Once individuals receive the diagnosis of a chronic illness, they often go through a spiral of information seeking. In response to a new diagnosis and a perceived information vacuum, many people talk to health-care providers, family members, and friends; they search the Internet relentlessly and read books and articles. Most people then reach a saturation point where they are overwhelmed with all the information they have encountered. They may be scared or distressed if the forecast for this illness is bleak, which can lead them to retreat and avoid any additional information about the illness. Others thrive on information and feel like they have a better grasp on their illness and what their illness experience may bring. This process is normal. It can ebb and flow over time and may vary greatly for each person and family.

For example, psychologist Suzanne Miller identified two groups of people who respond very differently to threatening health conditions like cancer.[6] She labeled them *monitors* and *blunters*. Monitors tend to be acutely sensitive and search for the negative and frightening aspects of a situation, while blunters actively resist acquiring information about the situation—the less they know the better. Are you a monitor or a blunter? Imagine that you are in the exam room waiting for the dermatologist to examine a suspicious mole on your shoulder. The nurse informed you the doctor is running late, so it will be ten to fifteen minutes before you are seen. Which of the following behaviors might you engage in while you wait?

1. You are on the Internet, searching for pictures of malignant moles.

2. You brought a novel in your backpack and begin reading it.

3. You are reading the pages you printed from a website about mole removal options.

4. You put your headphones on and relax to music.

5. You review the list of questions you prepared to ask the doctor.

6. You begin working on sudoku puzzles on your tablet.

If the odd-numbered items are activities you'd choose, then you may be a monitor. If you relate more to the even-numbered items, then it's possible you are a blunter.

Knowing your style matters because you may react differently to health-related information depending on your response style. For example, if your health-care provider calls and indicates that a test result was abnormal, a monitor will jump right to the thought that "I have cancer," while a blunter may not even return the call thinking that if it's serious, the nurse will call back.[7] If you are a monitor, you will likely want to ask your health-care provider to provide more information, estimates of risk, and seek reassurance that things will be okay. In contrast, if you are a blunter, you are likely less interested in reassurance and extraneous information, but if you recognize this tendency in yourself, you might tell your provider that it will help if he or she provides direct and honest evaluation of your situation. Then, warn them that your coping mechanism as a blunter is to be complacent, and invite your provider to make an extra effort to hold you accountable to the recommendations provided.[8]

One sometimes controversial source of knowledge is the Internet. This resource is clearly a mixed blessing in terms of access to health information. Thirty years ago, if patients wanted to gather information about a medical condition beyond general medical encyclopedias found in their public library, they would have go to university or medical school libraries to search the professional journals. Most of the information they would encounter would likely be above their heads unless they had medical training. Today, with the click of a mouse, we can find a plethora of health-related information. However, not all of that information is accurate and reputable or helpful. In fact, it can truly exacerbate already anxious reactions. Health-care workers speak of patients coming to them after first consulting "Dr. Google," and assigning themselves a diagnosis. So it is important to be careful to verify the content of the webpages we consult for medical advice.

How might this play out for a monitor versus a blunter? Monitors may seek out as much information as they can, particularly material that discusses the worst-case scenarios related to their illness. We know that a great number of illnesses are affected by the presence of stress, and it is possible that stress cycles into exacerbating symptoms or developing perceived symptoms that may not be present otherwise. It could also help prepare the monitor and equip him or her to better understand the possible scenarios. It can often go back to the meaning made about the information that is found. Blunters, on the other hand, may either avoid such searches altogether or practice selective attention and only attend to the more hopeful prognoses about their situation.

SUPPORT

Support comes in many forms. Some people seek support from family and friends, and others prefer to spend time alone to process newly learned information. Some like to participate in activities, and some like to create works of art. As previously mentioned, what works for one person doesn't necessarily work for someone else. There are no right or wrong ways to find and maintain support, as long as it contributes to an increased sense of well-being and a decrease in suffering. Finding the type of support that fits each person's own unique needs can be a very important part of attempting to manage and cope with chronic conditions.

Family and Friends

We don't exist in a vacuum: we are impacted by and impact those around us, whether they be family and friends or other larger social circles (church groups or health clubs). Building these systems into our coping plan can facilitate individual and collective healing around the diagnosis. Even if the illness itself cannot be healed, any potential social or relational complications that have resulted from the diagnosis can be improved.

People who care about your well-being can be great partners in helping you cope with illness. Through supportive conversation, family members, friends, and confidantes can help a person make sense of the illness, both what the illness means to them individually and what the illness means in the context of a family or friend group. For example, through supportive conversation, people can discover answers to questions such as, "What might have to change because of my illness? What can stay the same? How can we rearrange the family schedule to accommodate my treatment days or days when I feel really ill?"

Support Groups

Support groups come in all types and sizes. There are groups available through specialty care centers that encourage participants to discuss their experiences with illness such as cancer, MS, and Alzheimer's disease. There are support groups that are sponsored by community groups, where those with addictions come together to discuss sobriety-related challenges and successes. And there are online communities where people share experiences and information about a large variety of chronic illnesses. Thus, decisions about which group or groups to attend can be based on characteristics such as desire to meet in person or online, ability to travel to an in-person group, or desire to focus on overall wellness or illness-specific stressors. No matter which group you choose to attend, sharing experiences can truly help you to navigate many of the themes that people with an illness find in common. The shared experience that comes from connecting with others, either in person or via long distance, is validating and can help a person feel that they aren't the only one going through a particularly difficult set of challenges. Additionally, the opportunity to support others in the group can be rewarding and may contribute to a larger sense of purpose.

Therapy

Meeting with a therapist, whether individually or as a couple or family, can be a powerful tool to use when newly diagnosed with a chronic illness. It can also be helpful over the course of an ongoing illness experience. Chronically ill individuals and their families might get lost in the day-to-day management of the illness and may need help stepping back to see a full picture of their experience. Perspective is often gained when a therapist can help a family remember that the individual and the family are more than just the illness.

As elements of an illness shift and change, families may have difficulty navigating these changes. For example, if a family member is living with Alzheimer's disease, their potential deterioration over time will likely create changes in the way the family navigates their daily lives. A therapist can help this process by facilitating meaning-making and discovering how each patient can use their unique skills, strength, and support networks to create greater well-being in their own lives.

ACTION ITEMS

So what can we do with all of the information above? How can we actually implement some strategies into our lives that will help us cope with and manage our own chronic illness experience or our experience of a loved one's illness? At this point, we've discussed some the main challenges as well as several coping and management tools of living with a chronic illness. Now we would like to offer some simple action items.

1. Be Mindful

We can begin to take action by simply being mindful of our experiences. Being mindful, or paying attention to the present moment and accepting of what we are experiencing in each moment rather than thinking back to "before the illness" or ahead to "what might happen" with the prognosis, can be a very helpful coping mechanism.[9] Witnessing emotions and thoughts within the illness experience can allow a person to *respond* to internal processes (feelings and thoughts) instead of *reacting* immediately to external stimuli, such as that intimidating Internet article or the bad mood of a health-care provider. Being mindful can also be instrumental in helping to create meaning surrounding an illness experience, since it allows for connection with what is actually happening moment to moment. (See chapter 6: Mindfulness.)

2. Accept Emotions as They Arise

Medical family therapists McDaniel, Hepworth, and Doherty referenced several emotional themes felt by those battling an illness.[10] These authors observed that these emotional themes have been found throughout many of their cases and the cases in the book, regardless of the type of illness or age of patients. Many may find strength in not feeling alone in these sometimes perplexing emotional experiences, since some of the emotions felt may feel like polar opposites of one another. Some of these paths the authors include are denial versus acceptance, despair versus hope, isolation versus connection, and secrecy versus sharing.

While these pairs of emotions seem to differ greatly from one another, people can experience conflicting emotions simultaneously. For example, in a family where an individual has been diagnosed with cancer, family members may feel despair over the loss they feel over their loved one's diminished health. They may feel hopeless about a difficult prognosis. At the same time, the family may feel hopeful that their loved one will receive the best treatment possible and hopeful that the family will be able to support one other through the course of the illness. While there are no absolutes in that every patient will experience all of these emotions, comfort can be found in knowing that commonalities exist.

There are as many ways to manage these emotions as there are people on the planet. For example, in the community of persons with multiple sclerosis, individuals often say "I have MS, but MS doesn't have me." In other words, they have a chronic illness, but that illness doesn't define them, nor is it who they are (they are not their illness). This sentiment can apply to all people with chronic illness and can be an important way to remember that people are not solely their medical diagnoses or physical limitations. Each person is so much more: a mother, a brother, a lawyer, a writer, a friend, and so on.

3. Seek Support

Find support! It is extremely important to seek out supportive experiences during the onset of a chronic illness. If there is something that has worked well for someone in the past, they may benefit from using that particular support again. If you aren't sure what will work for you, use trial and error to figure out what helps you feel supported and cope effectively. Maybe going to a therapist is an important first step for some, while binge-watching Netflix with a sibling feels supportive to others. There are countless options. Try a handful to see what works!

Mariela's Experience

Mariela had been recently diagnosed with diabetes. Because her grandfather and uncle had both lost their sight from uncontrolled diabetes, she believed she would also eventually lose her sight. After her diagnosis, she began withdrawing from her family and spending a lot of time in her bedroom. She also stopped painting landscapes, which had been a favorite hobby since childhood. Since she believed she would lose her sight, she no longer had the desire to hone a skill that she felt she would ultimately lose the ability to use.

Mariela's husband and two teenage children became concerned about her well-being. One night, she threw away her paints and didn't leave her bedroom to join her family for dinner, and they knew they needed to do something to help her. They asked Mariela to make an appointment with her doctor so she could have the opportunity to ask questions and figure out if she would, indeed, eventually lose her sight.

During Mariela's visit with her doctor, she learned about ways she could care for herself that would make it much less likely to lose her sight. Her doctor also recommended a diabetes education class and diabetes support group. Through the class, Mariela was able to learn diabetes management skills, including exercise and diet strategies that could help her maintain her health. In the support group, she was able to talk about her fears, the changes she was making in her lifestyle, and her hopes for the future.

Through a combination of all of these supportive experiences, Mariela began feeling like she had more control over the course of her illness and felt better prepared to manage the fears and difficult thoughts that arose. She found that she was able to analyze her emotions and could then respond to her feelings rather than reacting by becoming anxious or experiencing overwhelming fear. Although she still has to cope with the various aspects of managing her diabetes and she still has concerns about her health, she feels that she is able to control pieces of her illness experience and feels that through the support of her family and medical provider, she has the emotional and practical resources she needs to help support her throughout her illness experience.

CONCLUSION

Every person determines their own unique way to cope with illness, based on their innate strengths combined with the strengths of people around them. They may choose to consult with family or friends. They may seek information through online forums. They may attend support groups and online chat support forums. Or they may decide that none of these strategies is right for them. Finding out what it means to adapt and what illness means in each person's life is a wholly unique endeavor. As is often the case in life, typically there is benefit in finding balance between what is suggested and what makes the most sense for you and your family. It is important to normalize your experience by figuring out what this diagnosis or illness means to you and those around you. There will be things you can control and things you cannot, so learning to adapt to what you must, and seeking support for the problems that will be more difficult to navigate is an important part of the process. It will be more critical than ever before to be in touch with *your* voice (knowing your body, what you need, and being clear and assertive in expressing yourself) and *your* experience, while still finding a way to bring others into that and sharing in those experiences. By staying in touch with your voice, you will more likely to be able to determine the best way for you to manage this new chapter of your life.

NOTES

1.   Susan Sontag, *Illness as Metaphor and AIDS and Its Metaphors* (New York: Picador, 2013), 3.

2.   Centers for Disease Control and Prevention, "Chronic diseases and health promotion," accessed October 14, 2015, http://www.cdc.gov/chronicdisease/overview/.

3.   C. S. Russell, M. B. White, and C. P. White, "Why me? Why now? Why MS?: Making meaning and perceived quality of life in a Midwestern sample of MS patients," *Families, Systems, & Health* 24 (2006): 65–81.

4.   J. Kabat-Zinn, *Full Catastrophe Living: Using the Wisdom of Your Body and Mind to Face Stress, Pain, and Illness* (New York, NY: Bantam Books, 2013).

5. Posttraumatic Growth Research Group, "What is PTG?" 2013, accessed October 14, 2015, https://ptgi.uncc.edu/what-is-ptg/.

6. S. Miller, "Monitoring versus blunting styles of coping with cancer influence the information patients want and need about their disease," *Cancer* 76 (1995): 167–77.

7. "Monitors and Blunters: Different Patient Coping Styles," Cancer Network.com, accessed March 2, 2015, http://www.cancernetwork.com/articles/monitors-and-blunters-different-patient-coping-styles.

8. Ibid.

9. J. Kabat-Zinn, *Full Catastrophe Living.*

10. S. H. McDaniel, J. Hepworth, and W. J. Doherty, "Medical family therapy with somaticizing patients: the co-creation of therapeutic stories," *Family Process* 34, no. 3 (1995): 349–61.

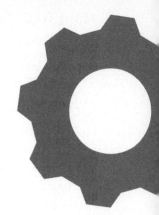

11 | THE ROLE OF MEDICINE IN YOUR LIFE

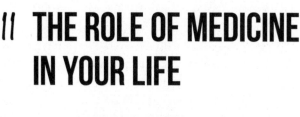

BY DAVID DUPREE, PHARMD

"WHEREVER THE ART OF MEDICINE IS LOVED, THERE
IS ALSO A LOVE OF HUMANITY."
—ATTRIBUTED TO HIPPOCRATES

DR. DAVID DUPREE, PharmD, *lives in Athens, Georgia, with his wife, Stephanie, and their family. He began his college education at the College of Southern Idaho with a focus on art and science. He took a break when he joined the US Army and served as an Arabic linguist in Operation Iraqi Freedom. David graduated from Idaho State University with a doctor in pharmacy. He currently works for the Rite Aid Corporation as a retail pharmacist. He has spent the last few years of his career focusing on clinical programs and training his peers.*

INTRODUCTION

Allow me to start by making a case for my profession and how we fit with other health and wellness professionals. Pharmacists, especially retail pharmacists, have to make themselves jacks-of-all-trades. Most people will see and discuss their health, lives, and concerns with their pharmacist more easily, and more frequently, than any other member of their health-care team. When a patient walks into the pharmacy with a small scab under her nose and complains of mild flu-like symptoms, we become frontline diagnosticians. In this case, the pharmacist noticed the connection between the small sore and the flu-like symptoms and told the patient to "March on down to the urgent care and get that MRSA infection taken care of." (MRSA, or Methicillin-resistant Staphylococcus aureus is a strain of staph bacteria that is resistant to most antibiotics, and while most infections are minor, some can be life threatening). This particular patient had her doubts about her pharmacist's advice but returned later that day with a prescription from the urgent care doctor and a lot of gratitude for a pharmacist who helped her with an early "great-catch" diagnosis that helped her get timely treatment.

A pharmacist also assumes the responsibility of on-the-spot amateur counselor and therapist, since patients are often at their worst, feeling exceptionally stressed, or just plain sick or tired when they call. When you are looking at a hundred different medications that say they will help your cold, and you have no idea which one to pick, we are happy to walk out and become merchandise experts. When a patient calls in because they have made a terrible mistake, we sometimes have the guilty pleasure of being the most important person in that individual's life during the duration of that phone call.

Here's an example: A patients calls in because very recently the mood has struck. The patient reaches into the nightstand and pulls out the trusty K-Y jelly. However, the patient is on the phone with you now because it was not K-Y jelly; it was another product. Needless to say, the product has lit a torch that will not go out! Any advice you can give to stop this inferno is priority number one in this patient's life and, "Please, please it needs to work and work fast!" A trusted pharmacist can be a nutritionist, a counselor, an authority on medications, and the best of us try to be friends and colleagues to our patients as well.

My primary focus for this chapter will be to discuss medications and how you can utilize them most effectively in your life. First, I would like to stress that medications can be a very important part of your overall health, but depending on the situation, they are not always the *most* important part. Your medication regimen is just a piece to the overall puzzle for keeping yourself healthy and happy. Having said that, there are some cases where distrust or avoidance of medications can lead to the worst kind of outcomes.

I spend a significant amount of my time at work helping patients manage their medications, so I take appointments for what is called medication therapy management services. I'm able to coordinate with patients, their physicians, other health-care professionals, and the pharmacy in order to get the best possible outcomes.

Let me show you why this service is vital and is one you might consider using more often: I came across a nice lady who wanted to sit down and discuss her overall health and, particularly, her medication management. The focus of the discussion became about strokes when I learned the patient had suffered two strokes in the last four years. This particular woman was distrustful of medications and just didn't like to take them. She had a history of high cholesterol, which contributed to her strokes. She had tried a medication that not only lowered her cholesterol but helped stabilize clots that had formed in her body. Unfortunately, she decided after a short time (without consulting her pharmacist or doctor) not to take this medication because she read some negative information about her medicine. She also wasn't on any form of blood thinner. The patient was doing everything she could to live a healthy lifestyle and thought that would be enough. Unfortunately, it took a second stroke to convince her that living a healthy lifestyle just wasn't enough in this case. There are times when a medication can save your life. At the same time, there are situations when medication can be harmful and unnecessary. We will discuss the role medication can play in order to be helpful to you and your family.

I hope to give some guidance and tools to help you avoid medications when possible, get the best results when medication is necessary, and discover ways to get the most out of your treatments. I will focus the discussion on four topics:

- know your medications
- understand that there is no magic bullet
- be honest
- avoid fads

KNOW YOUR MEDICATIONS

Have you ever tried to self-diagnose yourself using an Internet search? Have you searched for every reason there might be not to take a medication? When I say know your medications, it may not be in the way you are thinking. What I mean is know enough to be a part of the process, while allowing health-care professionals to be your guide. What do I mean by this? There is no way we can become something we are not. Let the physician be the physician and the pharmacist be the pharmacist, and do your best to be the educated patient who actively participates in their own health care. The most important thing you must know about any medication is what to expect when you take it. Allow me to illustrate:

A patient walks into the physician's office and gets the devastating news that his blood test reveals he has diabetes. The patient is now faced with an overwhelming list of changes that need to be made in order to prevent possible blindness, amputations, and premature death. Not the best day, by far. Now the physician reaches into her bag filled with all the choices available to help her patient manage this illness. He is so relieved there is a shiny new pill that will fix all of his problems. He leaves the office relieved, picks up his new medication, and goes about life in a normal fashion, never giving a thought to altering his diet or dealing with the sedentary lifestyle that is partly responsible for putting him in this position.

This is a bit of an oversimplification, but most patients leave the doctor's office without any idea of how well anything they are told to do will work. They focus on the solution in their pill bottle and often neglect the big picture of total health. On the flip side, some people look at the lifestyle changes they can make and neglect the fact that the medication is an important part of the process.

If you are diagnosed with type 2 diabetes, the current king of the castle is metformin. I don't want to get into too many individual medications, but metformin is so beneficial that I want every diabetes patient and everyone who knows someone with diabetes to be aware of a few tips. While metformin is currently the very best drug we have to offer diabetes patients, many people stop taking it due to stomach problems. Metformin can be taken at low doses and built up slowly. It can also be prescribed in an extended release formulation that sometimes reduces the stomach side effects. If you have diabetes, do everything you can to work with your provider in order to make it possible for you to take this medication. Even if you tolerate metformin well and get to where you are able to take it at the dose that will give the maximum benefit, the medication alone will not help you make large improvements if you don't address your overall health. I hope you'll read this book in its entirety so you can start to better define what you want in terms of overall health as you consider your nutrition, fitness, relationships, work-life balance, and other factors that impact your wellness *beyond* the use of medication.

An equally important question everyone should ask about their medications is, "How do I need to take them in order for them to benefit me?" Here's another true story: A couple came into the pharmacy looking for Plan B in order to prevent a possible pregnancy. The pharmacist showed the couple a product they could use but was cut off when he tried to give an explanation for how to use the product. They were in a hurry and had no time for any information. Even though the pharmacist tried to stop them, they rushed to the front and out the door after making their purchase. They were confident they knew how it worked and how to take it. Three months later, the couple returned very upset that the product didn't work. The product they bought had two pills. The pills were *both* meant to be taken by the female member of this party, but this gentleman took one for himself and then gave the other one to his lady companion. Some simple information on how this medication is taken was all this couple needed to prevent an unplanned pregnancy. Knowing your medications doesn't take a PharmD. It takes asking the questions you need and then *listening* to the advice given. You'll need to know these five important things about any medication:

1. What is the medication used for?

2. What is the expected result?

3. What are the reasons to stop taking this medication?

4. How often is this medication taken?

5. How does this drug fit into the overall picture of my personal wellness?

Most medications have somewhat modest results when taken perfectly, but when taken any other way, they have no positive effect at all, so it's important to be informed and then to follow instructions carefully.

UNDERSTAND THAT THERE IS NO MAGIC BULLET

I'm going to start this section by discussing the closest thing available to a magic bullet that has been discovered to date: vaccinations. I will also try to dispel some of the negative publicity that comes along with this topic. In 1998, Dr. Andrew Wakefield and several other coauthors published a study that linked vaccinations to autism. The study was based on falsified data and was completely fraudulent. However, this study has been blasted on radio waves, on television, and in magazines for years and helped drive the antivaccination mentality. I encourage all of my patients to stay up-to-date on all vaccinations available, and I am personally up-to-date on my own vaccinations. I encourage everyone who doubts the effectiveness of this medical achievement to take another unbiased look at the pros and cons. I would hate for one of your little ones to be a victim of measles, for example, like some of the individuals affected in recent outbreaks. This is a completely avoidable situation that comes in the form of a simple vaccine.

Another topic that everyone is hungry to discover a magic bullet for is obesity. This is a topic that puts information in a fire hose and then sits us all down for a drink like we can soak it all up and figure it all out. We are bombarded with ways to lose weight. Products are constantly coming to market that promise weight loss, but the reality of the situation is there is no easy solution. Many over-the-counter products will present studies that show the product is a success. However, many weight loss studies are skewed in ways that hide the true result. In the *best-case scenario*s, some of the prescription products will lead to a weight loss of around five to ten pounds over a period of a year or more. The weight is difficult to keep off, and the medication can come with serious side effects. In the *worst-case scenarios*, many weight loss products help sustain a little weight loss over a few months but usually plateau or even lead to mild weight gains when studied for longer periods of time.

The drive to use these products is extremely strong because we all know how hard it is to lose weight and want an easy fix. But if you've learned anything from this book, you should have learned this: an easy fix is a rarity in health care, if it exists at all. Wanting something to work really badly will not make it a reality. The best way to lose weight requires multiple lifestyle changes, patience, and consistency, and in my professional opinion should usually not include over-the-counter or prescription medications.

Some people might look at this topic and think, *Well, if there is no perfect solution, why should I take my medications at all? If my medicine helps only a little bit, what is it good for?* Many people with a chronic disease have a goal of one day living a medication-free life, and if patient do everything they can to live a healthy lifestyle, this is sometimes possible. But the reality is, in *most* situations and for *most* people, good health is a struggle and a lifelong process. There are many bumps in the road, and each of us stumbles. If the goal is to get to the point where you no longer need blood pressure medication for instance, then pulling the plug early is the worst way to try to get there.

This concept seems simple, but people do it all the time. I've been helping a patient for a while; I manage her blood pressure medication. She updates me on her appointments and changes in therapy. She was so happy one day when she came in and said the doctor said her blood pressure was just perfect and that she is doing great. A few months later, I noticed she hadn't picked up her medication in the last few months, so I called her up. She said she was doing so well she didn't need medication anymore and decided to stop her blood pressure medication on her own. I asked her to please come into the pharmacy so we could check her blood pressure and see how she is doing. Not surprisingly, her blood pressure was highly elevated, which confused the patient. She took information from the doctor the way she wanted to hear it. She stopped doing what was working and decided on her own to stop taking a medicine she didn't really want to take to begin with. She had been changing her lifestyle in the many ways recommended, but didn't understand just how much the medication was helping to get her that perfect blood pressure. She still has the goal to get off her medication but will wait for her physician to tell her when it is time. Again, wanting something badly enough does not always make it happen. Medication is not the only answer to most health problems, but in most cases it is a very important piece of the puzzle.

BE HONEST

It is important to have the most accurate information in order to help someone improve an aspect of their health. The problem is, people lie. We all do it. More than anything, most of us do not want to admit that we aren't doing what we know we are supposed to do. Every patient I talk to wants to say they take their medication perfectly, eat the healthiest diet, exercise all time, are happy and healthy, and never go against doctors' orders. Many of them have convinced themselves that this is true no matter how I ask, but most will come clean eventually. Many of us disappoint ourselves in various ways and have a hard time telling others about these situations. I no longer even ask patients if they are taking their medication the way it has been prescribed, because the answer is always yes. Even if I'm looking at a sheet of paper that says you only pick up your diabetes medication 50 percent of the time, the answer is still, "Nope, I take my medicine."

From experience, I know it works better to have a discussion on the difficulties of taking medications and challenges patients face. I have a patient who brings in a bag, and it's a big bag. It is chuck full of all the medication he needs to take. Even after going through them and trying to weed a few out, it is still a big bag. Many medications will only work well if they are taken every day or even multiple times a day. The pharmacy team now helps this patient by filling up his weekly medication boxes for him. The challenge of taking all his medications in the way that they will benefit him is not an easy one, so he has been wise to allow us to use our expertise to help make it simpler. Taking medication improperly sends hundreds of people to the hospital every day. Your pharmacy team can help keep that from happening, but only if you are honest with us, which may mean being really forthright with your pharmacist about what is working and what isn't.

Medication adherence is a constant problem for patients and providers. If you can't stand your little orange pill because it makes you pee too much and you have a hard time making it to the restroom, don't be afraid to say that very thing. If you remember all your morning doses but never take your midday doses, let us know. Many times, we can change the formulation of your medicine, and then you will only need to take a morning dose. If that stupid little pill that costs way too much each month is just not in your budget, let us try to find something that you can afford. If you don't know why you are taking medication X and just don't think you want to anymore, come talk to us about it. Many medications have known side effects that limit their use. However, some of these medications are still the best available treatment for a particular ailment. A warning and a few things that can be done to minimize these side effects will help many patients stay compliant.

Many people have various reasons why they don't want to take their medicines. Many of these reasons are unjustified and simply require a little more information or an alternative. The problem we all face as patients and providers is that oftentimes people won't be honest about what they are doing. Some patients will require two or three medicines for the same condition. Other patients will be put on multiple medications because they never took the first medication properly. This is difficult to discover, unless the patient is completely honest with the provider. I can't tell you how many times I've heard, "That medication just doesn't work for me," or, "I'm allergic to this medication." I often find that it doesn't work because maybe you aren't taking it, or what you thought was an allergy was something everybody feels, and if you just make a small adjustment, that side effect might go away. This line of complete honesty should be encouraged to follow all of us through this journey we call life. Keep in mind that I *want* to help you not just because it's my job but also because it gives me real pleasure to be of service to another human being. It's the reason I chose a service occupation. If your pharmacist isn't service-oriented, find one who is.

AVOID FADS

Here's the first thing you need to know about fads: newer is not always better. Although I'm a pharmacist, I have my own "medical trust issues" based on bad experiences I've had in my life. I've had three separate surgeries that did not go as smoothly as expected. One left me with pneumonia. Another resulted in an uncomfortable experience with anesthesia, and a third left me with a massive hematoma that took months to heal. The result is that I have a real fear of going under the knife. When I was in the army, stationed at Fort Gordon, Georgia, I suffered a hip and back injury. I spent months trying various therapies with limited success. I was approached about a new surgery, but when I heard the phrase *new and experimental*, I said, "No, thank you very much" to both the surgery and to the military and decided to take a new career path.

We all are excited about new technology, new movies, or new anything really. This is almost always the worst kind of attitude when it comes to new medications. I'm not saying new medications are bad. Many times they are very good. What I am saying is many times the new medications are unnecessary and, most of all, extremely expensive. Most of the therapies that are considered the gold standard of treatment are not new at all. In fact, the opposite is true. They are heavily studied, with known outcomes and expectations. New medications are thoroughly studied as well, but the long-term outcomes data and especially all the possible future effects are still a big mystery with a newer drug. In many cases, a new medication will come out that is *not* going to be the next big thing but rather is just another version of something that was already available on the market. You will find the "combo products," which combine a few old medications to be taken together. These are packaged up and sold at top dollar as "new" drugs.

It is always best to have an honest discussion with your provider about the best choices available. Try to avoid using an advertisement to guide your choices in treatment. Most of the best medications do not need advertising because all the physicians already know to use it. This topic leads into another fad in medications that is usually wrong as well: more expensive is always better.

When I met with one patient recently and he told me how much he was spending each month for his health care, I asked if I could try to save him some money. He looked at me like I was crazy and said, "I'm not worried about the cost; I just want the best." I told him I would be happy to tell him if each of his medications were the most appropriate for his conditions. Turns out most of them were not. He had a list of expensive medications, but for his conditions the best treatments were skipped over. The patient had a really hard time believing medications are not always like everything else. There is no "you get what you pay for" type of thinking when it comes to treatment. I was finally able to convince this patient that not only was I going to help him get on what works the best for most people, but that was also going to save him hundreds of dollars.

The next myth is a bit of a hot spot for people: natural is always better. Let me start by saying I am not one of those providers who is against alternative health care. There are all types of remedies that can help patients that are considered "alternative care." I take my recommendations from both American and European guidelines, as well as other credible sources. I recommend many natural and alternative forms of treatment. But I've discovered that most consumers who favor alternative treatments have an "us versus them" mentality when it comes to natural versus more conventional medicine. You might be interested to know that a host of medications behind the counter are produced wholly from natural sources. The big difference between vitamin and herbal therapies and prescriptions is not *where* the chemicals they are made from come from. Rather, it's a case of *how thoroughly* the chemicals derived from various sources are studied.

In order for a prescription to come to market, it must be proven effective. Natural treatments, unfortunately, do not have that same burden. This is where the confusion starts for most health-care professionals. The data to support the use of many supplements is lacking. Even when studies have been performed, they are not held to a standard that would fulfill all the requirements that most health-care professionals rely on to make a recommendation. This is the reason many natural treatments are really just a shot in the dark. Aside from testimonials, there's no hard data for a physician to review prior to recommending a nonpharmaceutical product. That lack of "hard evidence" may make it difficult for a physician to be confident in a recommendation for most alternative therapies.

It's also important to note that there are supplements and vitamins that can be harmful. Natural does *not* always mean safe. It is a good idea to try to get the best information available, and, if yours is a serious condition, my advice is to lean toward the evidence-based medicine that has passed the rigors of testing and retesting.

CONCLUSION

The amount of information on this topic is vast, but I want you to begin today to be a more active participant in your own health care. It is important to remember that pharmaceuticals have been a great benefit to society. We currently have treatments for conditions that would have amounted to a death sentence only a few years ago, but we still have a long way to go in understanding total health. Relying on a treatment for all that ails us and forgetting the role those treatments have in our overall lives would be a mistake. Your medications are just one tool in the health-care belt we all have access to. Don't rely on just one tool when the job of keeping ourselves healthy and happy requires so many.

 ## ACTION ITEMS

1. Stay adherent (your medications will only work if you let them).

2. Be honest (with yourself and your providers).

3. Get immunized (it is a shame not to utilize such a powerful tool).

4. Get educated (know what your treatments are expected to do).

Good luck and happy trails on your path to better health!

SECTI⚙N
4

OUR RELATIONSHIPS

"Piglet sidled up to Pooh from behind.
'Pooh!' he whispered.
'Yes, Piglet?'
'Nothing,' said Piglet, taking Pooh's paw.
'I just wanted to be sure of you.'"

—A. A. Milne (The House at Pooh Corner,
Methuen & Co. Ltd., 1928)

12 FAMILY RELATIONSHIPS AND HEALTH

BY RICHARD B. MILLER, PHD, & JEREMY YORGASON, PHD

"THE EVIDENCE REGARDING [MARITAL] RELATIONSHIPS AND HEALTH INCREASINGLY APPROXIMATES THE EVIDENCE . . . THAT ESTABLISHED CIGARETTE SMOKING AS A CAUSE OR RISK FACTOR FOR MORTALITY AND MORBIDITY FOR A RANGE OF DISEASES. THE AGE-ADJUSTED RELATIVE RISK RATIOS ARE STRONGER THAN THE RELATIVE RISKS . . . REPORTED FOR ALL CIGARETTE SMOKING."[1]

RICHARD B. MILLER, PhD, *is a professor in the School of Family Life at Brigham Young University. After receiving his bachelor's degree in Asian studies from BYU, he earned his PhD in sociology at the University of Southern California. His research focuses on the importance of healthy marital relationships on societal well-being, including the impact of relationship conflict on adult and child functioning in the United States, Taiwan, and China. He has published research articles in numerous journals, including* Journal of Marriage and the Family, Family Relations, Journal of Marital and Family Therapy, International Journal of Aging and Human Development, Journal of Comparative Family Studies, Family Process, *and* Journal of Health Psychology.

JEREMY B. YORGASON, PhD, *is an associate professor in the School of Family Life and director of the Family Studies Center at Brigham Young University. His research interests focus on later-life family relationships, with an emphasis on marriage and health, grandparent-grandchild relationships, and preparing for retirement. His work has been published in several professional journals, including* Families, Systems, & Health; Family Relations; Journals of Gerontology, Series B: Psychological and Social Sciences; Journal of Family Issues; Journal of Aging Studies, Journal of Applied Gerontology; *and* Research on Aging. *He received his PhD from Virginia Tech in human development, with an emphasis in marriage and family therapy. He is a licensed marriage and family therapist in the state of Utah.*

The quote at the beginning of this chapter suggests there is significant research that has documented the fact that marital conflict and other forms of marital distress do more to harm an individual's overall health than smoking cigarettes does. Does that surprise you? Did you realize that marital problems are such a significant risk factor for poor health? Unfortunately, even though researchers are very aware of the strong link between marital problems and poor health, little attention has been given by government officials, policy-makers, insurance companies, health advocates, and the general public to reinforcing the important role that healthy marital and family relationships play in the well-being of adults and children. The two are so significantly linked that we've decided to make the topic the focus of an entire chapter of this book! We'll discuss two significant aspects of relationship distress, family illness, and marital distress, and discover ways to overcome the negative impacts of each.

MARITAL DISTRESS AS A RISK FACTOR FOR HEALTH PROBLEMS

The good news is that most married couples are happy and satisfied with their relationship. They generally enjoy being together, they love each other, they are able to successfully deal with conflicts and disagreements, they communicate well, and they are generally satisfied with their sexual relationship. However, the bad news is that a sizable proportion of couples are unhappy. For example, a large national study of married couples found that 31 percent of them reported being unhappy in their relationship.[2] They reported low levels of positive emotion, frequent communication difficulties, an inability to resolve conflicts, and dissatisfaction with the quality of sexual and nonphysical intimacy.

Physical Health Problems

Think about that for a moment! From a public health perspective, if 31 percent of the married population were experiencing an increased risk of heart attacks or an increase in diabetes rates, that problem would probably be considered an epidemic that would warrant major attention from the government, public agencies, and the private sector. And as we will see in this chapter, these couples who experience relationship distress *are* at serious risk for health problems. These problems include poor physical and mental health.

Let's take a look at some facts:

- One of the authors is completing a major review of the research articles that have examined the link between marital quality and physical health. His research team has found 152 articles, and they consistently show that poor marital quality is predictive of poor physical health.

- Specifically, poor marital quality has been linked to health problems, such as the following:
    - heart disease
    - chronic fatigue syndrome
    - tooth cavities
    - ulcers
    - obesity
    - hardening of the arteries
    - flare-up of rheumatoid arthritis symptoms

- Negative marital interaction (arguing and criticizing) has a bigger effect on physical health than positive marital interaction (showing support, affection, and encouragement). In other words, the effects of arguing (toward poor physical health) is greater than the effects of affection and support (toward good physical health).

Why is the quality of marital relationships a significant risk factor for physical health? Research suggests that there are three main "pathways" between poor marital quality and physical health.

1. Adults in low-quality marriages are more likely to experience stress. Indeed, in many situations, marital conflict is chronic, which creates chronic stress. In turn, stress (especially chronic stress) is a serious risk factor for health problems.

2. Adults in low-quality marriages are more likely to engage in risky health behaviors. For example, they are more likely to eat unhealthy foods, have inadequate and low-quality sleep, abuse alcohol, smoke, and misuse prescription drugs. Each of these poor health behaviors are linked to poor physical health.

3. Marital conflict has been linked to negative physiological changes, such as decreased immune functioning, increased blood pressure, and increased inflammation. These negative biological processes are all related to poorer physical health.

Mental Health Problems

Marital distress is also a significant risk factor for mental health problems. One of the authors has conducted a series of studies that has examined the effect of poor marital quality on depression. The findings are clear that men and women who are in low-quality marriages are significantly more likely to experience depressive symptoms, as well as be diagnosed with major depression. The reason for this is that in low-quality marriages, spouses are less likely to provide support to each other, and they are more likely to interact with one other in hostile ways. Being in a relationship that is characterized by daily low levels of social support and high levels of hostility puts a person at risk for depression. Looking at mental health more broadly, in addition to depression, research shows that poor marital quality is a risk factor for anxiety disorders, such as social phobia posttraumatic stress syndrome and generalized anxiety, as well as bipolar disorder.

Children

It gets worse! Not only does poor marital quality have a negative effect on spouses, but it also puts the children at significant risk for health and social problems. Children who grow up in homes that are characterized by frequent arguing between the parents are more likely to experience poor health, depression, and anxiety. They are also more likely to struggle in school, experience problems associating with their peers, have low self-esteem, have eating disorders, get in trouble with the law, and have an out-of-wedlock teen pregnancy.

The truth is that children do not do well when they are raised in a war zone. Amazingly, some children are resilient, and they are able to survive growing up in a hostile and stressful environment. But most children are at a significant risk when they grow up in a home where they experience significant conflict. Children are sensitive to the atmosphere in the home, and they experience stress when there is a lack of peace and harmony between their parents. Interestingly, it just isn't arguing and fighting among parents that has a negative effect on children. Some parents don't argue openly; rather, the conflict is more covert, characterized by angry distance, "the silent treatment," and passive-aggressive behavior. Children who grow up in these homes also struggle with their physical health, mental health, and social competence.

WHEN ILLNESS IMPACTS FAMILY RELATIONSHIPS

We have been talking about how family relationships, and marital relationships in particular, have an impact on physical health. The truth is that the connection between family relationships and health can go the other direction as well. Health challenges have different impacts on our family relationships depending on the type and severity of an illness, how long the illness is expected to last, and if it is life threatening.

Put simply, there are three main illness situations that impact families:

1. Acute daily illness symptoms such as a cold, headache, sore muscles, minor injuries, broken bones, and other health challenges that are short term.

2. Chronic illness or ongoing health problems, such as illnesses common in later life (arthritis, for example), auto-immune diseases (multiple sclerosis or MS, for example), and illnesses that require medication regiments and long-term medical involvement (diabetes, for example).

3. Illnesses that pose a significant life threat, such as the leading causes of death in the United States. These might include cancer, cardiovascular diseases, chronic obstructive pulmonary disease, and stroke.

When individual family members are affected by daily acute illnesses, they might not have their typical positive mood (they are grumpy!), and, as a result, they might engage in more conflict with other family members. Further problems might result from not getting enough sleep, being in pain, or simply being irritated because of not feeling their best. Family members—including parents, children, siblings, and spouses—are often relatively patient with each other during acute illnesses because the duration is known to be relatively short.

Chronic health problems can take a greater toll on family relationships than acute ones. Chronic illnesses are often hard to diagnose, taking weeks, months, and sometimes even years to figure out. These types of health problems often result in big life changes, including having to stop or change employment; changes in who does what jobs around the house; and having ongoing medical visits, bills, and prescription medications. Due to life changes from chronic illness, families facing such challenges often experience financial strain, caregiving burdens, and sometimes a pileup of various other challenges.

For example, one of the authors has a daughter who has a form of low-functioning autism. Her developmental disabilities make it impossible for her to care for herself and function in society. Family life in this household has been drastically changed because of her disability and the parents' responsibility to care for her. With other children in the family, the challenge has been to try to have a "normal" family life in the context of very non-normal circumstances. They have had to work to accommodate her daily needs, while providing a home life that allows the other children to have opportunities to grow and develop in normal ways.

Life-threatening illnesses bring some of the same challenges to families as chronic illnesses, but they also add unique demands, such as intense medical treatments and abrupt changes in life plans. Such illnesses can have a forceful impact on family relationships because they bring a sense of urgency and a realization of the reality of mortality. Families are often forced to go into emergency mode to meet these illness demands.

For example, one of the authors' parents had been married for almost fifty years when his father was unexpectedly hit by a major stroke that left the father disabled. He was paralyzed on the left side of his body, which made it difficult for him to walk, and he had great difficulty speaking; he also experienced cognitive decline, which affected his ability to think clearly and to remember things.

In an instant, the parents' relationship changed. His mother was abruptly thrust into a full-time caregiving role. After being partners for fifty years, his mother now had the responsibility to take care of his father and to make the major decisions in their relationship. The relationship changed—even simple tasks that had always been taken for granted required adjustment. For example, it was weird to see his parents pull up in the driveway with his mother driving. Because of his father's disability, the marital relationship had to adjust in order to accommodate this new health dynamic. The father's condition gradually worsened, and her caregiving responsibilities increased, until he died nine years later.

Circumstances That Influence the Impact of Health Challenges

A number of life circumstances influence how health challenges impact families. The first is age at the time a family member becomes ill. Acute illnesses are expected to come and go throughout life, yet chronic and life-threatening conditions have a stronger impact, or are less anticipated, when they occur during childhood, adolescence, and even into middle adulthood. In later life, health challenges can still present major challenges, yet they are expected to some degree. One way to think of this is that an illness can be "on time" or "off time." An "on time" illness might be a major illness in later life, when it is *expected* that older adults will start facing serious health problems. On the other hand, an "off time" illness might be diabetes in a ten-year-old boy or multiple sclerosis in a thirty-five-year-old woman. These "off time" illnesses are more stressful on families because they require the family to make significant accommodations at a time in life when families typically don't have to deal with these kinds of issues.

Access to medical and community resources can be very helpful when dealing with illness. Medical resources might include a physician and nurses you trust, having insurance coverage, and having appropriate treatment available. Although some medical resources are subject to your circumstances, others can be sought out, such as learning all you can about an illness.

Finally, which family member is ill can impact family circumstances. When a mother or father is ill and there are still young children in the house, there is an immediate impact on necessary daily tasks in the home, such as meal preparation, cleaning, and shopping. There may also be an impact on finances if the parent that is ill has to stop working. When a child is ill, at least one of the parents often becomes heavily involved, and any other children and a spouse relationship might receive less attention. In the end, there are factors that can impact how illness affects families, and knowing about these can help families to view their particular challenges in a different way.

The Silver Lining

While most people wouldn't ask for a severe or ongoing illness, there are some families that grow closer together as a result of one family member being ill. Specifically, parents draw closer to their children as they serve and care for a family member's needs. Siblings learn a special way of caring for each other when one is ill or has a disability. Spouses providing care for one another may become closer to each other as a result of the illness. All family members can assist as caregivers to their loved one, and in this way develop a special bond that comes only through this type of service. In essence, families can become resilient and close when they work together to overcome difficult challenges.

What Can Be Done to Strengthen Families When Illness Strikes?

When people become ill, families can do the following to lessen negative impacts and strengthen family relationships, despite the challenges:

1. *Use "balanced coping."* Pay appropriate attention to an ill family member while also acknowledging challenges of other family members. With the demands of caring for an ill child, it is easy to focus too much time and energy toward that child, which inadvertently may lead to siblings feeling resentful. It is a constant balancing act to meet the extraordinary needs of a severely ill child while also meeting the needs of the other children. The important thing is to be mindful of the issue so that you are constantly trying to balance the two sets of needs. Not being aware of the issue creates blind spots that may lead to benign neglect and subsequent resentment.

2. *Balance support with autonomy.* Balance support and involvement for ill family members with appropriate levels of autonomy. You want

them to feel connected and part of the family, but you also want them to feel that they are able to make appropriate treatment choices about how the illness and the surrounding circumstances should be handled. For example, honor the ill family member's preferences about how much information about the illness is shared with others outside of the family.

3. *Expect and adjust to ambiguity.* There are times where sure outcomes are unknown, especially regarding health diagnoses and treatments. Learn to live happily despite ambiguity, or not knowing how things will be in the future.

4. *Remember that illness is an experience, not a personal characteristic.* Try not to let illness become the center of your identity and relationships. Acknowledge illness, but maintain aspects of personhood that aren't related to illness. William Doherty, a prominent marriage and family therapist who has specialized in health issues, has said, "A family needs to make a place for the chronic illness in the family, but they also need to put the illness in its place. Just like an extended visit from an unwelcome relative, you need to accommodate them, but you don't need to let them stay in your living room. Rather, you can have them stay in a back bedroom, where they aren't the center of attention. So it is with chronic illness in families."[3]

5. *Grieve losses.* Allow grieving when hopes and dreams change due to illness.

6. *Keep a positive attitude.* Try to keep a positive attitude, and look for the good in your circumstances. Sometimes looking outside yourself by providing service to others helps you stay positive.

7. *Avoid "protective buffering."* Protective buffering occurs when family members avoid difficult conversations with an ill family member. In the short term, this often detours around highly emotional topics. However, in families, long-term healthy relationships work best when difficult illness topics (treatments, prognoses, and long-term side effects) are addressed along the way.

WHEN MARITAL DISTRESS IMPACTS FAMILY RELATIONSHIPS

Recognizing the important connection between marital relationships and health, what can we do to help people be happier and healthier? Looking first at how low-quality marriages are a risk factor for physical and mental health problems, let's explore two different strategies for helping marital relationships to be strong.

1. Prevention

The first strategy is prevention. When one of the authors was much younger, he was a distance runner, and one of the lessons that he learned from years of running in races was that it was easier to *keep up* than to *catch up*. Likewise, it is much more effective and efficient to keep a marital relationship strong than to have to go through all of the pain and effort of repairing a marriage that is broken. This brings up another metaphor: car *maintenance* is less costly and more convenient than car *repair*. Indeed, the principle of prevention is widespread in the health-care industry. Insurance companies encourage their customers to get regular dental check-ups and to have their teeth cleaned because they have learned that dental check-ups reduce the number of costly cavities and more serious dental problems. Likewise, mothers and fathers are encouraged to take their babies to the doctor for well-baby check-ups because the *prevention* of problems with babies is cheaper and more humane than the *treatment* of problems.

So how can we maintain strong marriages and prevent marital problems? Here are three suggestions: First, and perhaps the most important thing, is for couples to be mindful and conscientious about maintaining the richness and vitality of their relationship. Our world today is increasingly hectic and stressful. The demands upon us and our children continually increase, leaving us with less and less time to nurture our relationships. Unfortunately, the demands of our careers and parenting children often take precedence, and the one thing at the end of the week that we too often ignore on our to-do list is the time that we had planned to spend with our spouse. Over time, a continually neglected marital relationship loses its life and vitality. What was once a strong relationship filled with love becomes a hollow and lifeless entity. Much like a flower, love and relationships need constant nurturing. Just as water and sunlight enable a flower to grow and blossom, marital love requires spouses to nurture the relationship. What is considered nurturing in one relationship (chocolates, flowers, jewelry) may differ from that of another relationship (movie night, dinner at a restaurant, or a long walk together). Thus, it is important for spouses to learn what their spouses find nurturing and to conscientiously provide that nurturing. In sum, marital problems can be prevented by each spouse making a conscious effort to nurture their relationship.

Second, couples can read good books together about how to maintain strong marital relationships. This experience can provide excellent information about the principles of successful relationships, give spouses opportunities to discuss the principles they are learning, and provide them with a common set of concepts and principles that help the couple be on the same page. The challenge is that while there are hundreds of marriage books on the market, many of them simply spread bad information and marriage myths. Based on our experience working with clients and on our scholarly research, we can recommend any of the four following titles:

- *The Seven Principles for Making Marriage Work: A Practical Guide from the Country's Foremost Marriage Expert* by John Gottman (New York: Three Rivers Press)

- *Hold Me Tight: Seven Conversations for a Lifetime of Love* by Sue Johnson (New York: Little, Brown & Company)

- *Reconcilable Differences: Rebuild Your Relationship by Rediscovering the Partner You Love—without Losing Yourself (Second Edition)* by Andrew Christensen, Brian D. Doss, and Neil S. Jacobson (New York: Guilford Press)

- *Fighting for Your Marriage: A Deluxe Revised Edition of the Class Best-seller for Enhancing Marriage and Preventing Divorce* by Howard J. Markman, Scott M. Stanley, and Susan L. Blumberg (San Francisco: Jossey-Bass)

Third, couples can benefit from attending marital enrichment or marital education workshops. There are many opportunities for couples to participate in classes or weekend retreats where they learn principles for healthy marital relationships. These classes and workshops also often provide the couples with opportunities to practice the skills they are being taught. The research on these marital enrichment activities shows that they *improve* relationship functioning and they *reduce* the probability of divorce. Consequently, they are a good investment for couples to make.

Just like books about marital relationships, couples need to be careful that they only attend high-quality workshops or classes that are based on sound, research-based principles. There are many high-quality marital enrichment programs available, but be certain that you research your options and attend a workshop that uses a curriculum that you can actually find and verify on the Internet. Also, be wary of workshops that promise too much. Just like financial workshops that promise to "make you a millionaire in only three hours" are probably scams (or at least a waste of time), so, too, are workshops that promise to teach you "three easy steps to having a perfect relationship."

2. Treatment

Perhaps your marital relationship is broken and in need of repair. The good news is that research on marital therapy (also called marriage counseling) has demonstrated that, overall, it is effective in helping couples relieve their distress and improve the quality of the relationship. Specifically, research indicates that marital therapy helps couples reduce their level of anger, develop more positive feelings toward each other, increase their positive interaction in the relationship, and improve the quality of their communication.

So how do you know if you need marital therapy? Many couples have the ability to repair their distressed relationship without outside help. However, there are times when things get so bad that even highly skilled couples are struggling and can't seem to make things better. Like sports, relationships seem to have momentum; when the momentum is good, everything seems to go well. However, in the case of distressed couples, the momentum is negative and everything seems to go badly. Even well-intentioned interactions seem to go sour. It is almost as if the couple is flying an airplane, and the airplane takes a dangerous nosedive. If, no matter how hard the couple tries, they can't pull out of the nosedive, it is time for them to see a marital therapist. In other words, if, despite their best efforts to repair their relationship, they are unsuccessful, then it's time to seek outside professional help.

If you decide that you want to see a marital therapist, it is extremely important that you find a good one. Unfortunately, that is not as easy as it may seem. There are many, many counselors who advertise marital therapy; however, few of them have actually received specific training in doing marital work. The truth is that couples therapy is very specialized and complex, and it takes sustained, advanced training in order to gain the skills necessary to provide effective therapy. As an analogy, a dermatologist may be an expert at treating skin conditions, but you wouldn't go to that doctor for open-heart surgery; rather, you would seek out a cardiologist who has extensive training and experience. Likewise, you want to do your homework and find a therapist who specializes in doing marital therapy and who has received extensive training in it. The Internet provides a useful tool to help you do your research on possible therapists.

One last piece of advice is to not wait too long before seeking marital therapy. Both of us are marriage and family therapists who specialize in working with couples. One of the sad situations that we encounter is when couples come in for therapy after their relationship has deteriorated to the point that it is almost beyond repair. I have often found myself wishing mournfully that these couples had come to therapy when there was still some life in their relationship instead of waiting until it is practically too late. So, if you need marital therapy, don't delay! Just like cancer, the sooner you get treatment, the better the prognosis!

NOTES

1. James S. House, Karl R. Landis, and Debra Umberson, "Social relationships and health," *Science* 241, no. 4865.

2. M. A. Whisman, S. R. H. Beach, and D. K. Snyder, "Is marital discord taxonic and can taxonic status be assessed reliably? Results from a national, representative sample of married couples," *Journal of Consulting and Clinical Psychology* 76 (2008): 745–55.

3. William Doherty (speech, Kansas State University, Manhattan, KS, 1992).

13 BECOMING WHOLE AND HEALING CONNECTIONS

SIMPLE WAYS TO TRANSFORM YOUR MARRIAGE

BY FALINE B. CHRISTENSEN, PHD

"A DEEP SENSE OF LOVE AND BELONGING IS AN IRREDUCIBLE NEED OF ALL PEOPLE. WE ARE BIOLOGICALLY, COGNITIVELY, PHYSICALLY, AND SPIRITUALLY WIRED TO LOVE, TO BE LOVED, AND TO BELONG. WHEN THOSE NEEDS ARE NOT MET, WE DON'T FUNCTION AS WE WERE MEANT TO. WE BREAK. WE FALL APART. WE NUMB. WE ACHE. WE HURT OTHERS. WE GET SICK."[1] —BRENÉ BROWN

FALINE BATEMAN CHRISTENSEN earned her PhD from Texas Tech University with research that developed understanding of divorce and marriage through the eyes of women of faith, using a unique online questionnaire and gathering significant information regarding their beliefs, expectations, and experiences with marriage, divorce, deity, family, faith communities, and therapy. Faline has worked with many individuals, couples, and families to help them heal their relationships and find more happiness and balance in all aspects of life. She has taught undergraduate and graduate students, and she supervises new marriage and family therapists toward licensure. She is the manager of The Woodlands Center for Couples & Families in Texas (TheWoodlandsFamilies.com). She lives with her husband and provides a great place for her children and grandchildren to have lengthy visits in the lovely community of Montgomery, Texas.

Editor's note: It is important to note that although the chapter is directed to married couples, the principles could easily apply to committed partners, engaged couples, and many types of relationships.

INTRODUCTION

Several years ago, my husband and I, along with a good friend of ours, took a five-day canoe trip down the Missouri River, following eighty-five miles of the Lewis and Clark trail in Montana. We have enjoyed doing active outdoor things together in our marriage, like trail riding, hiking, camping, and tubing, but we had never done a canoe trip together. We both thought it would be fun! Also, I had an idea of facilitating "extreme marriage counseling" with couples participating in a challenging yet beautiful environment, and I wanted to try it out first before investing further in the concept. The couples-counseling-in-a-canoe idea never came to fruition, but some of the lessons from our experience on the river have stayed with me.

The Planning and Preparation

The planning for the trip actually began several months before we finally launched our canoe into the Missouri river current. We spent hours answering our questions: When is the best time of year to go? Where should we start and end? What do we want to eat? How much work do we want to spend on cooking? What supplies will we need? And on and on. The preparation included increasing our physical workouts so that we would have the stamina and staying power for the entire journey. Quitting was *not* in our plan for us, no matter what!

While it's important to plan and prepare to have a successful short canoe trip, it is even more important to plan your future life with your spouse. Get to know each other really well. Explore and buy into each other's dreams and goals. Find out each other's needs and wants. Treat each other like best friends. Prepare. Get ready for the lifetime commitment of marriage. Practice communicating clearly and listening well. Be positive. Encourage each other. Be flexible. Know that things don't always go as planned, and be prepared for that. Plan for the next day, or for the next month, just as you would for the next portion of the river. Planning is never done!

The Paddling

If you want to arrive at your planned destination, whether it's a particular spot on the river to camp for the night or a happy, satisfying, and soul-fulfilling marital friendship of many years' duration, you both will need to paddle pretty much constantly and as a team. This is not a one-person responsibility. It takes two. It means working together, using your shared strengths, and coping with your shared weaknesses. Also, the map you consulted in the planning and preparation stage doesn't tell you everything you need to know. At one of our end-of-day planned camping spots, we couldn't tell from the map, but right there in front of us was a little inlet that required paddling the canoe backward into it. I can tell you from experience that it's not easy to follow directions from your spouse when you can't see where you're going!

After several attempts, we finally succeeded in getting to shore where we secured the canoe. You won't always get it right the first time in your marital relationship. There will be highs and lows. Share both the high points and the low points together. After all that coordinated paddling—and we became pretty good at it!—we then had to carry all our stuff up a steep incline to our campsite. Difficult! But wow! The view of the river from up there was breathtaking! Sharing the hard times and the good times is part of what makes you a successful couple.

It's always a choice. You can choose to paddle together or not. But I can promise you that merely drifting does not take you where you want to go.

The Rapids

In every marriage, like on every big river, there will be trials and challenges. You will not always agree on what to do. If your canoe gets hung up on a rock, one of you might think it's best to get out of the canoe and push, while the other might promote staying in the canoe and pushing off with the paddle. Some differences and challenges you know from the beginning. Sometimes you may foresee a problem. Other times there may not be much warning or preparation.

The Loading and Unloading

Marriage, and canoe trips, consist mostly of the daily tasks of life. In marriage it may be chores, discussing the budget, and cleaning up messes. On the river it's the daily unloading at night and loading in the morning. Heavy cast iron pots and pans, heavy coolers and boxes of food, heavy tents and sleeping bags . . . at the end of a long day of canoeing, everything is heavy! And then carrying it up (always up!) to our campsite for that day. We have to get it all out of the canoe because we need it for the camping part. The canoe has to be taken out of the water also, or it might become unmoored and be lost to the river in the night.

In marriage, there are daily rituals that keep couples connected and provide emotional safety and security. The hug and kiss, the foot rub, the "unpacking" of the day with the talk of friends and partners, or sharing the household tasks are things couples who stay together do pretty much every day. This is hard work sometimes, and it's also necessary. The hard part is that you will each see things differently, and you will have different priorities. But those are good things also. Both of your perspectives are valuable in making shared decisions.

The Camping Part

On the river there is sweating. At the campsite there is dirt. There are mice and other critters. There is no toilet, clean or otherwise. There is cooking.

Everyone is hungry. A fire needs to be built. The cooking and camping sites need to be cleaned up. There is no shower. It gets cold at night. You try to stay warm. All of these things are true, *and* they are part of the journey you accept in exchange for the opportunity to see that amazing night sky, those awesome white cliffs filled with swallow-dwellers, and the soaring eagles. In the marriage, there are two very different people. Support each other in each of your dreams and goals. Show your love for each other, and savor the high points of your journey together!

The Marriage Journey

In my experience, people marry expecting to stay married for the rest of their lives, just as we picked up those paddles and stepped into the canoe for the duration of the journey. As adult humans, we are hardwired to seek connection with someone who loves us as we are, someone who listens to us and understands us, someone who appreciates us and makes us feel important, someone we can count on to be there for us no matter what, someone who believes we are special and number one in his or her eyes.

At the same time, it's probably not surprising to learn that many couples become less satisfied in their marriage after the birth of their first child. In addition to the demands of parenting, other pulls of modern married life—work, cell phones and other electronics, social and entertainment media, and even friends and extended family—contribute to "marital drift" away from the excitement, hope, and promise of the wedding "launch" day, and into strong and dangerous currents we don't necessarily understand or even, sometimes, notice until damage has been done to the couple connection.

Current research by Gilad Hirschberger and others indicates that when couples feel strongly connected to each other, both husband and wife are more likely to be satisfied and happy in their marriage, even when there are life challenges.[2] We yearn for a strong connection with our spouse. There is a real drive to seek physical and emotional closeness with our spouse. There is a desire to know that you matter immeasurably in your spouse's life. It is our nature as humans to need to trust that our spouse will respond with love and security. We all feel a need to be close to and connected with that other person. Indeed, there are physical and emotional benefits when you have that sense of connection with your loved one.

- You are less likely to experience depression, anxiety, and mental illness.
- You feel more confident.
- You tend to be more assertive in all areas of life.

- You feel more resilient when under stress.

- You are more open to new information and you are better at learning.

- You are better able to cope with the uncertainties in life.

- You recover faster from illness.

- You heal faster from wounds and from surgery.

- You have a reduced risk of heart attack, but if you do have one, you will heal faster.

James Coan, PhD, has been conducting research since 2006 using hand-holding as a variable, and he came to this conclusion: feeling closely connected to your spouse is the most efficient way of dealing with and coping with distress. His research has also demonstrated that the brain doesn't distinguish between pain and distress you are experiencing and the pain and distress your spouse is experiencing. In other words, if your spouse is hurting, you hurt too. Dr. Coan explained that we hold hands to "send each other's brains a signal," that says "I am here with you."3

I am here with you. This is a powerful message that implies additional strong messages: "You can count on me," "I have your back," "You matter to me," and "I will always be there for you."

After many years of working with couples as a marriage counselor, I would say that being able to trust in your spouse in this way is exactly what you were seeking before you found each other. And yet, if you've been married for any length of time, it's likely that one or both of you may have noticed, and even commented on, not enough quality time with each other, having sex less often and with less passion, fewer long talks, and more unresolved arguments. Maybe you feel like you aren't paddling together as well as you used to. Maybe you don't want to get to the dangerous rapids unprepared, and you're hoping to learn what to do to deal with it. Maybe it feels like you are already in the rapids and if you don't do something quick, your marital canoe will capsize.

I'm glad we went on that canoe trip. It was challenging. The setting was absolutely stunning. It is great to be able to paddle through a rough stretch of water and look back with laughter at the mistakes we made. At the end of the journey, it felt wonderful to know I had a partner I could count on in every way, every day, and he knew he could count on me in the same way! Sue Johnson, PhD, (author of *Hold Me Tight*) has stressed that this close emotional connection "is not just friendship, or social support. It's a relationship that's life or death, essential to survival."4

Healing and Attachment

We are born with the survival need for close emotional connection with the adults who love us unconditionally. As infants we start life completely helpless. We need loving adults to feel an attachment to us and care enough about us to feed us, protect us, and keep us clean and warm. We need to be held and patted and stroked. We need the comfort of soft words and gentle touching when we feel hurt or scared. We need them to play with us and laugh with us. We need loving adults who are totally "into" us. We need to be loved, wanted, and cared for just as we are, in all of our stinkiness. Human infants can't take of themselves. They sometimes die if their needs, both physical and emotional, are not met. Don't get me wrong. We don't always get our needs met. Realistically, the adults we rely on—our parents—are not always responsive to our needs. None of us have perfect parents. But even if our parents are pretty wonderful, none of us escape childhood unscathed, because parents aren't always there. They aren't always nearby or accessible or attentive. They leave us to go to work. They do things without us. They make unjust decisions and impose unfair punishments.

It isn't always something parents have control over. Tyler is the second of five children. When Tyler was seventeen, his father had been engaged in non-military assignments in the Middle East for eight years, coming home only once a year to spend three weeks with his wife and children on a dream vacation. Though Tyler interacted with his father regularly on Skype and email, he didn't believe that his father really knew him or cared about him as an individual. In Tyler's view, his father saw him as "just one of the children." When his father came home permanently, Tyler struggled. He wanted to feel close to his father, but he was critical of him and blamed him for being so unavailable all those years. He was distressed. Tyler had "learned" that he couldn't count on his father to be there for him.

We are hardwired to seek emotional connection throughout our lives. Recent research looking at adult attachment behavior would indicate that Tyler, as an adult, would turn to his spouse to meet his attachment needs of feeling close, being accepted, being heard and understood, feeling important, and feeling appreciated, and she would turn to him.[5] That's what we do as adults. We like to be close physically with our spouses. We don't like to be separated from each other. We seek comfort and assistance from one another. From the security of this special bond, we are able to handle challenging situations with confidence.

We also know that the way we connect with one another is influenced by attachment patterns. Attachment theory was developed by John Bowlby and has grown into a robust science, helping us understand how people connect or how people have difficulty connecting. In general, those that have a secure attachment style will seek connection with others in a healthy manner. In a couple relationship, a secure attachment is built on the ability to emotionally share with one another the good, the bad, and the ugly. We share our struggles, concerns, worries, achievements, joys, and excitement with those we love. As we share, we trust that the other partner will not use the vulnerability and information shared against us; rather, we trust they will seek to understand, value, and appreciate the sharing. The attachment creates a bond that protects and soothes during hard times while adding to the joy and peace of the good times.

Some couples engage in an ambivalent attachment pattern. We sometimes call this the "push-pull pattern," in which the couple chases each other or runs away in a push-pull fashion. A spouse may "chase" another spouse by reaching out to them and trying to connect while the other distances. When the other spouse stops distancing and begins to accept the connection, the other spouse now begins to run away as the other one chases them. The vicious cycle! They are never apart; they are never together. An ambivalent attachment pattern is based on a need to connect with a fear of full connection due to getting hurt in the past. Fortunately, the work of Sue Johnson and others have led to some breakthrough approaches to help couples with ambivalent attachment patterns form secure attachments. *Hold me Tight* by Sue Johnson (one of the books listed at the end of the chapter) is a great introduction to ways to help couples form more secure bonds.

My goal for this chapter is to teach you and your spouse some simple tools that will help you strengthen and heal your marriage. In this chapter, we will look together at five spheres within marriage. In each of these spheres, there are many opportunities to connect and reconnect with each other. These tools are about securing attachment with your spouse in order to provide a safe haven for both of you during times of high need or distress when you desperately need to know that you can reach your partner. You can safely seek aid and comfort from each other. You will have the power, when you put these ideas to work in your marriage, to heal past and current emotional wounds in your connection with each other. Your secure attachment will thicken and grow, toward wholeness in your marriage.

1. THE PLANNING & PREPARATION

Be Best Friends

Many couples seem to expect that since they love each other, everything else will just fall into place. However, planning and preparation need to include developing a strong friendship with your spouse. Current research provides evidence that people who are married to their best friend report their satisfaction level is double that of other couples.[6]

Best friends know each other. They are interested in each other's hobbies and talents. It's good for your marriage to share your interests with each other, and develop new interests together.

Donna loved music. She played the piano and she liked to sing. She enjoyed symphony orchestra concerts, choral programs, and marching bands. Bill was interested in other things. He hunted, he rode his horses, and he enjoyed taking care of his calves and chickens. They both liked to read. Bill thoroughly enjoyed listening to Donna sing and play piano, and he went with her to concerts. Donna supported Bill's annual hunting trips, and she learned to ride horses with him. Sometimes, they read each other's books. In the last few years they have done some traveling together. Donna really enjoys visiting new places, and Bill really enjoys being with Donna, so it works out for them.

Best friends enjoy each other. Be playful with one another. Laugh with each other. Steve and Lori (2015) started their relationship as friends. She didn't feel pressured to try to impress him. In fact, she told me that she wasn't romantically attracted to him at first. They spent months getting to know each other. They shared interests in tennis and track, and he often joined her in those sports. Lori liked to do unexpected things just to see how Steve would react. Once she wore black lipstick on a date, and he went along like everything was normal. They played jokes on each other, like the time Steve showed up at her door with a paper bag over his head. They had fun together. She often said that the thing that really appealed to her about him was that he made her laugh. You could adopt this for a success slogan in your marriage: "The couple that plays together . . . stays together!"[7]

Best friends are good to each other. Many years ago, I became friends with Jeremy and Corrinne, newlyweds of a few months. They shared with me a very wise philosophy that they had implemented in their marriage. They promised each other that they would never say anything bad about the other person to anyone. They are still happily married after almost fifty years of keeping that promise to each other. So be kind. Only speak good things about each other, to everyone, every time. Do nice things for each other. You don't need a reason, and you should not expect anything in return. Although if it is reciprocated, be grateful out loud. Take notice of your spouse's "favorites." If something is important to your spouse, recognize it and honor it, even if it's not important to you.

Your best friend encourages and supports you. As BFF ("best friend forever"), you need to be the number one person in your spouse's "amen corner." Remind your spouse of his or her best qualities, especially when he or she feels vulnerable. Be the number one defender of your spouse to everyone. If someone talks negatively of your spouse, defend him or her. Katie and James had been married five years and had a small child. Katie was sometimes unsure of herself as a mother, and James always pointed out the good things she was doing. In fact, he never let anyone criticize her, including his mother! Be the lead cheerleader of your spouse. Share in your spouse's happiness. It's always more fun to be happy together. Celebrate in your spouse's success. If your spouse has accomplished something (even a small something), congratulate and cheer.

Best friends are reliable. They are dependable. They are "there" for their spouse. Make every effort to come through with what you said you would do. In marriage, this is not always easy or simple. There is an episode from *Grey's Anatomy* where a woman fell into a sink hole; her husband fell in after her and stayed with her through the whole ordeal. He even amputated her leg to free her from a car that had fallen in also. When she woke up from surgery, she was extremely distressed that her husband wasn't there. When they brought him in from his hospital room, her face lit up, and she said, in tones of wonder and awe, "You stayed!"[8] Some may say, "That's not realistic. It's just a TV show." Yet, there are husbands and wives who do what best friends do, and stay, even when it's hard. Sylvia developed Parkinson's disease just a few years after she and Stanley started enjoying their retirement. During the inevitable decline of her mind and body, Stanley never stopped caring for her and trying to make her comfortable. Parkinson's is a disease of gradual and unrelenting loss, and over several years, Sylvia lost the ability to talk and to think. They lost the ability to be intimate, and finally, near the end, she lost her ability to swallow. There was a time, a few years before Sylvia died, when Stanley felt like he had lost his wife, and he considered getting out of the canoe. He thought about several options, but ultimately he did what a best friend would do: he stayed. He told me later that he had no regrets.

2. PADDLING

Make Time and Take Time Together

Many couples are starved for time to spend together due to competing work schedules and multiple responsibilities. Try nourishing your marriage over meals. Eating is something everyone has to do, and going out for a meal with your spouse can be enjoyable and inspire fun memories. Carla and Simon developed a tradition of going to different restaurants almost every time they went out to eat.

But you don't have to leave the house to bond over food. When you make a point of eating together at home, it's a way to have quality time with each other, which is an essential element in well-connected marriages. Quality time while eating together needs to be intentional. For example, James and Rebecca started a habit of sharing one thing they were each grateful for before they start eating. They both say that thinking through your day, searching for the positive, helps you know just how lucky you are. It's a good idea to protect your meal time together, by agreeing there will be no discussing conflicts and no using electronics. In the movie *The Story of Us*,[9] they had a nightly ritual over dinner of sharing their high points and low points of the day. When we started doing this over our meals, someone's high or low point often led to a longer and fascinating discussion, and we got to know each in new and interesting ways.

To add another dimension, you could try cooking together. Making time for making meals together is a sweet gesture that sends a message to your spouse that they are important to you. Take turns preparing, or share the cooking. Learn the stories behind his favorite foods. Find out why she prepares something a certain way. For instance, Donna learned that Spencer's mom always washed up as she went, and that's why Spencer did the same.

Take a look at the greetings and good-byes in your marriage. Make sure that before you say good-bye in the morning you have learned about something that your spouse plans or expects to have happen that day. Be interested. Be curious. This will tell your spouse, "You matter to me!" If you come home first, make an effort to welcome your spouse when they arrive home. If you come home second, go find your spouse to say hello and reconnect. As soon as you can, turn that greeting time into a fifteen-to-twenty minute stress-reducing conversation for both of you. Find some way to convey your fondness and thankfulness toward your spouse every day. Long hugs and short hugs. Hold each other. Touch each other. Even grab each other in playfulness. Kiss each other before going to sleep. I love how John Gottman (author of *The Seven Principles for Making Marriage Work*) described this good-night kiss: "Lace your kiss with forgiveness and tenderness."[10]

Josè and Maria came to me because they no longer felt the spark in their marriage. They were both busy. They told me they used to enjoy four-wheeling together, but now Josè would go with his brothers and friends, and Maria would spend time with her family and friends. They just didn't spend any time together. They still liked each other, and they missed what they used to have. Their homework was to pull out the calendar and find places to add couple time. This may seem too easy. Please don't ignore this just because it's easy! Do this together. Pull out the calendar for the week. First, put in the items that have to happen, such as work, church, appointments, and so on. Then, with your marriage as prime importance, put "couple time" on the calendar. It may start with only two to three hours a week, but make it a priority.

Support Each Other's Hopes and Dreams

First you have to know the hopes and dreams of your spouse. You could ask, "What is your fondest unrealized dream?" or "If you could do or be anything, what would it be?" Both of your hopes and dreams are important. Then set goals together. Early in the first weeks of their marriage, Michael suggested that he and Michelle create a goal poster. They discussed specific things they wanted to accomplish together. In their case, they both wanted to finish their college degrees, have children, and travel to Australia. Then they printed pictures that represented those goals and glued them to a poster board and hung it in their bedroom. They have added new goals to the poster over the years. Sometimes it is a goal for just one of them, but they both take ownership of every goal. They take time about three or four times a year to plan and discuss their progress. When they reach a goal, they celebrate.

3. THE RAPIDS

When the Going Gets Tough . . . Keep Going

Listen to each other, *especially* when it's hard! It can be really hard when you are having a disagreement. Yet this is a critical time to listen with your eyes. Notice your spouse's body language. Notice the cues that tell you your spouse is getting angry, frustrated, or anxious. Learn your own and your spouse's triggers—those things that send you or your spouse over the top. I invite couples to use a strategy honed by Kent McDonald, clinical director of Sandy Counseling in Sandy, Utah. I ask couples to sign a commitment to use a planned time-out in those situations. Time-out for couples has two purposes. First is to calm down. Second is to develop at least one possible solution to the problem or disagreement that led to the time-out. A planned time-out should never last more than one hour. Do healthy things to calm yourself down. Think of at least one possible problem-solver. At the end of your planned time-out, come together, reconnect, and talk about the possible solutions you both came up with.

Here is another way to handle differences. Think of a time when you were having, or were in the beginning of, a disagreement (a fight, argument, conflict, or difference of opinion). Up goes the radar scanning for danger, and you go on alert—"She's going to start yelling, I just know it!" "He's about to put me down!" "There she goes, rolling her eyes at me!" "He's mocking me!" You are expecting name-calling, put-downs, sarcasm, and sneers. Then, out come the guns, ready to shoot, and duck!

The mind may be going crazy, or it might go numb. The tension goes up. The listening goes down. In this high-alert state, the heart rate goes up, muscles get tight, faces get red, jaws tense, hands clench, and it is hard to notice anything but the emotional danger signals. Maybe one spouse will say or do something to reduce the tension, lighten things up, and try to keep the negativity from going out of control. Hans winks at his wife, Ashley, and she cracks up, and the tension is gone! Julie says to Richard, "I'm feeling flooded here. Can we take it slower and softer please?" My personal favorite is asking for a do-over: "I think I really messed up here. Could I try and say this a different way?" And my husband pauses, and says, "Yes. Please." And his expression says, "Thank goodness! We're not going to have a fight!"

John Gottman calls these "repair attempts" the secret weapon of happily married couples.[11] If a couple has a strong friendship, they get good at recognizing and sending these repair messages. However, when the couple's relationship is heavy on the negativity side, they may not even be able to notice any positive signals over the cacophony of the emotions in the moment. I believe that taking the time to learn these repair statements and then practice using them in times of disagreement in your marriage is one of the most valuable things you can do for your marriage. In every situation, *how* you respond is key to getting through unscathed.

4. THE LOADING & UNLOADING

The Little Things Are the Big Things

"It's the little things that matter." That's what Barry, the contractor who remodeled my bathroom, said when he learned I was writing this chapter. And he's right. He was talking about putting a built-in bench in the shower area, which makes shaving legs easier for the woman. After all, "It makes her happier!" What this comment means here is that it's important to make decisions with your spouse in mind. Be thoughtful about what is important to your spouse. What will make him comfortable? What will make her smile?

Every marriage is filled with the daily tasks of life: laundry, dirty dishes, paying the bills, cleaning up after pets, and lots of cleaning and putting away.

Whether you do these things together or separately doesn't matter so much as that you are both engaged in it. After all, you both live there. Going "fifty-fifty" or keeping track of who does the most doesn't really work in marriage. At various times, one or the other will need "more." Look at those times as an opportunity to make that day a little better for your spouse.

Build in rituals that you both value. Many couples have incorporated spiritual or religious rituals such as attending religious services or having couple prayer together. One way to cherish and nourish your marriage is to be thankful in prayer for your spouse and express some of the reasons for your gratitude. Joanne and Carl make the bed together every morning and consider it "starting the day out right." Ron and Kerry look forward to their nightly reading to each other. They have read many books together. If you don't have any special rituals yet, then, as a couple, think about rituals in your extended families or among your friends and selectively borrow rituals and make them uniquely yours.

Expand Your Perspective

One of the most difficult chronic situations to deal with is when couples each have narrow perspectives. Robert and Susan argued incessantly about whose interpretation of a recent event in their marriage was the "right" one. They called each other liars, when really they were only describing the view from their corner of the relationship. I said to them, "Suppose you were both looking out the same large window but toward different directions." When I asked them each to describe what they saw, each description was accurate to the view available to the one describing, but it certainly did not agree with the description of the view available to the other person. One saw a home in the distance. The other saw a busy road. Both views were accurate, yet each was only a part of the whole picture.

There is a way to get out of this toxic mire. Think about what you know about your spouse and how that might affect how they see things. Your spouse may not actually be doing anything wrong, just different from what you would do. Remember, there is no divine way to _____ (fill in the blank): no divine way to select a new lamp; no divine way to fold towels; no divine way to mow the lawn, and so on. We get stuck trying to be right, and what we really need—connection, closeness, safety, to be heard—gets missed. Practice stepping into your spouse's shoes and looking through your spouse's eyes.

What Job Did Your Spouse Hire You to Do?

Clayton Christensen (author of *How Will You Measure Your Life?*) developed a theory around business success that also applies to marriage success.[12]

Just as companies focus more on what they want to sell their customers than finding out what customers really need, we think more about what we want in our marriage rather than what is important to our spouse. What is needed is empathy. You need to seek deeply to understand what problems your spouse is trying to solve by "hiring" you to be a spouse. Your spouse may not be able to state clearly what those problems are, so you need to put yourself in your spouse's shoes, in your spouse's chair, and in your spouse's life. Warning! The jobs that your spouse is trying to do are probably very different from the jobs that you think he or she should want to do. Have you noticed that we tend to give our spouse what we want to give, and what we have decided our spouse should want to want? This looks like selfishness to me!

Cynthia thought of herself as helpful. The way she helped her husband Mike was to point out how he could do better, how he could get a better job, how he could be more successful. She was pretty pleased with herself for being so helpful and always full of ideas to improve things. She expected Mike to thank her for helping him, but instead Mike was very upset with her. She was stunned. She didn't know what she had done wrong. However, Mike wasn't looking for her advice and critiques. He wanted her encouragement and support. He wanted her to be uplifting and positive. He wanted her to believe in him.

It can be hard to get this right in marriage. Even with the best of intentions and love, we can profoundly misunderstand each other. We assume things. And yet, when husbands and wives figure out the jobs that their partner needs to be done, and then they do it well, they both fall more deeply in love, and they create an abiding emotional connection.

5. THE CAMPING PART

Increase the Positives

What you focus on expands in your view of things. It's like you turn on the "zoom in" feature. If you focus on what annoys you about your spouse, all you will see are reasons to be annoyed. On the other hand, if you focus on what you love about your spouse, you will be filled to overflowing with love. Always try to see the best in your spouse. And then notice it out loud. If you do this, you will likely discover that what you comment on, what you praise, and what you appreciate out loud is what you will get more of. Love and happiness both flourish in a positive environment.

Let's be honest with ourselves here. It's not easy to stop being critical, or to stop focusing on the flaws. If our spouse ignores our requests or complaints, we are likely to up the ante and start criticizing, blaming, and name-calling.

Sometimes we are critical because we have learned in our lives that what we do is never good enough, and we criticize ourselves. Then, because we have trained ourselves to notice what is wrong or missing, we focus on our spouse's flaws too rather than appreciating his or her wonderful qualities. Then there are people who criticize because they believe they are being helpful, as in, "I'm pointing out this behavior you should change because I only want the best for you." Frankly, this is *not* helpful in marriage! Let's face it. Criticism doesn't make a marriage better. It doesn't feel good. You don't like to be around someone who is criticizing you. Your spouse doesn't enjoy it when you criticize.

As you replace criticism of your spouse with words of kindness and an attitude of gratitude for your spouse, you can expect that you will refind purpose in your marriage, and your life together will become more satisfying, meaningful, and fulfilling.

Love and Affection

Many people have heard something about love languages. We can thank Gary Chapman (author of *The Five Love Languages*) for turning his observations of couples into a useful tool for understanding what your spouse needs to feel truly loved by you. According to Dr. Chapman, we all have ways of expressing love that are familiar and comfortable for us. You and your spouse may have very different ways of expressing love and affection. Mary Kay Ash (founder of *Mary Kay Cosmetics*) told about the weekly tradition that her husband Mel Ash began before their marriage. Every Thursday until he died he gave her a gift. Sometimes it was a handmade card, a lovely rose from the garden, or occasionally it was something more expensive. Every week she found a gift from him. It was his special way to show her he loved her.

The most important thing to know is that we all need to feel loved and appreciated by our spouse. Be generous with your expressions of love. Lots of hugs and kisses. Lots of sincere compliments. Do things for each other. I have told many husbands that vacuuming through the house might be the best beginning of foreplay they have tried in a long time. Watch and observe how your spouse shows love to you. That may give you a clue about his favorite love language. See if you can figure out how to say "I love you" to your spouse in her love language.

When There Is a Violation

There are times when safety needs are violated in marriage. Some examples include a betrayal where a spouse feels like a stranger, physical violence, criticism and contempt, or emotional or physical leaving. While these are significant violations, experiencing one does not necessarily mean that the marriage has to end. I do have hope for difficult cases such as these. I have seen enough couples change that I know it is possible, even if I can't accurately predict the outcome of a particular marriage. Sometimes couples who have been greatly disappointed in their marriages think they are the only ones in an imperfect marriage. When they feel alone and disconnected from each other, they lose hope for healing. Some of them divorce, but possibly many more continue to stay miserable and disconnected.

I am an advocate for happy, connected couples. What I want you to know is that there are couples who face big challenges and betrayals. They work through them. They develop better patterns. And they end up building something better from the wreckage. The route to healing includes, in part, developing a healthy pattern of reliable and predictable accessibility, responsiveness, and emotional expression over a period of time. The principles that have been described here will definitely be useful in this situation. This is a situation when you probably need the help of a well-trained marriage therapist.

Taking Action for Your Marriage

Change doesn't occur until somebody does something. It only takes one person in a marriage doing something differently to start both of you down a whole new exciting path. You have been introduced to many ideas that, taken together, can transform your marriage. Just because they are simple doesn't mean they are easy. This is not a checklist to get through but a long-term project for marriage enrichment and healing.

1. *Be best friends.* Take a close look at your attitude and behavior toward your spouse. First of all, ask yourself, do you think like a best friend toward your spouse, or not? Decide on one way you can be a better friend to your spouse, and follow through with this for thirty days. Notice what feels good about this new way of thinking about and treating your spouse.

2. *Make time together.* Raise the priority of your marriage by giving it dedicated time on your calendar. Marriage needs consistent attention and care. You might notice what gets more of your time and attention, and rethink what is most important in the big picture. Select one activity at a time that will nourish your marriage. Talk about what you like about it and what you might change to make it more useful to your marriage.

3. *When the going gets tough, keep going.* Practice a different way of handling differences and conflict in your marriage. The goal isn't always to fix the problems but rather to keep talking. If there's a disconnect, then reconnect.

4. *The little things* are *the big things.* Think about things from your spouse's perspective. What matters to your spouse should matter to you. Make sure you know what matters. Let go of the need to be "right." Let yourself remember that there are many possible ways to do anything. It can be enlightening to think about some of the benefits of doing things the way your spouse does things. You could let your spouse know what you are thinking.

5. *Increase the positives.* Give at least one sincere, wholehearted compliment to your spouse every day for a week. Notice any differences, both in your spouse and in yourself. Do it for one more day. Then do it for another day, and another. Look for what is special about your spouse. Be grateful for those qualities in your spouse. Value the contributions your spouse makes in your life. Of course, this all has to be honest and genuine and from your heart. No faking. No being phony. Just notice these positive qualities. Try to tell your spouse what you notice and what you sincerely appreciate about him or her. Just find one positive thing each day. Ignore all flaws and shortcomings.

Since you are reading this chapter and you have come this far, you are probably someone who enjoys reading self-help books, and you are likely on the lookout for ways to improve your marriage. Your spouse is probably not just like you in this regard. When one spouse starts talking about new ideas and new patterns, the balance of the marriage can be disrupted. It's like changing the dance steps right in the middle of the music. Stepping on toes. Having to watch your step. Two left feet. When I became a marriage therapist after thirty years of marriage, I had learned a lot of ways to improve my marriage and I wanted to do them all NOW! My husband and I would agree that it wasn't easy. What I have learned is to make one change in myself at a time and *always* be respectful of my sweetheart.

You can do something new without announcing it in advance. For example, if you have been in the habit of sleeping through your spouse's departure in the mornings, you can set your alarm to wake up before your spouse leaves. Make it pleasant for your spouse. You don't want to mess too much with their usual morning routine, but you can express gratitude, and you can show affection. Do it every morning for a week. You can let your spouse know that you enjoy those "good-bye moments." If you think your spouse has enjoyed this time also, then you can suggest that you do this regularly.

If you are the *very* unusual couple who is reading this chapter together, you still will want to make just one change at a time. Explore these new ideas together. Try them out with an honest and sincere trial of at least several weeks. Talk about the change you are making. Improve it to fit your needs. Make it yours. Make it better.

CONCLUSION

I picture in my mind the many couples who started their marital journey on the river of life. They were filled with high expectations, anticipation, and dreams. Months and years later, some things have changed, and other things have stayed the same. With illnesses, addictions, financial problems, and sometimes multiple marriages behind you, you may still yearn for that soul-filling deep emotional connection with a spouse who will be there and stand beside you in the midst of life's challenges. My hope is you will find some answers here for emotional and physical well-being in your marriage and family relationships. I'm with you on this river! Let's all keep paddling!

BOOKS I LIKE FOR IMPROVING MARRIAGE RELATIONSHIPS

Fighting for Your Marriage: Positive Steps for Preventing Divorce and Preserving a Lasting Love by Howard Markman, Scott Stanley, and Susan L. Blumberg (San Francisco: Jossey-Bass, 2001). You can improve your communication and conflict resolution skills by reading and practicing the principles presented in this book.

Hold Me Tight: Seven Conversations for a Lifetime of Love by Sue Johnson (New York: Little, Brown & Company, 2008). Through stories of real couples from Dr. Johnson's practice, enlightening advice, and helpful exercises, you can learn how to nurture, protect, and grow your marriage toward a lifetime of love.

How Can I Forgive You? The Courage to Forgive, the Freedom Not To by Janis A. Spring (New York: HarperCollins, 2004). This healing book offers step-by-step, concrete instructions that can help you make peace with others and with yourself.

Take Back Your Marriage by William Doherty (New York: Guilford Press, 2001). This book addresses three major stressors on marriage-parenting stress, career stress, and outside interest influences and offers practical solutions to these problems, as well as how to resist family, friends, and even marital therapists who may undermine or threaten your marriage.

The Seven Principles for Making Marriage Work by John Gottman (New York: Three Rivers Press, 1999). The framework to create and maintain a "sound marital house" is explained and illustrated with numerous examples, enlightening quizzes, and marriage-enriching exercises.

NOTES

1. Brené Brown, "Want to Be Happy? Stop Trying to Be Perfect," accessed October 23, 2015, http://www.cnn.com/2010/LIVING/11/01/give.up.perfection/.

2. G. Hirschberger et al., "Attachment, marital satisfaction, and divorce during the first fifteen years of parenthood," *Personal Relationships* 16 , no. 3 (2009): 401–20.

3. J. A. Coan, H. S. Schaefer, and R. J. Davidson, "Lending a hand: Social regulation of the neural response to threat," *Psychological Science* 17, no. 12 (2006): 1032–39.

4. Sue Johnson, *Hold Me Tight: Seven Conversations for a Lifetime of Love* (New York: Little, Brown & Company, 2008).

5. R. C. Fraley and K. E. Davis, "Attachment formation and transfer in young adults' close friendships and romantic relationships," *Personal Relationships* 4 (1997): 131–44.

6. S. Grover and J. F. Helliwell, "How's life at home? New evidence on marriage and the set point for happiness," NBER working paper no. w20794 (2014), available at SSRN: http://ssrn.com/abstract=2545179.

7. L. C. Schade, "To stay together . . . play together. Uniting Couples to Strengthen Families," March 31, 2015, https://drlorischade.wordpress.com/.

8. T. Phelan and J. Rater, "Free Falling," *Grey's Anatomy*, episode 149, directed by R. Com (Hollywood, CA: Prospect Studios).

9. *The Story of Us*, directed by R. Reiner (West Hollywood, CA: Castle Rock Entertainment, 1999).

10. J. M. Gottman and N. Silver, *The Seven Principles for Making Marriage Work* (New York: Three Rivers Press, 1999), 22.

11. J. M. Gottman, "Relationship repair checklist," 2010, https://pbs.twimg.com/media/Bo5xcn-CUAAnjRT.png:large.

12. C. M. Christensen, J. Allworth, and K. Dillon, *What Job Did You Hire That Milkshake For? How Will You Measure Your Life?* (New York: HarperCollins, 2012), 112–15.

14 SPIRITUALITY AND HEALTH

BY PATRICK R. STEFFEN, PHD; JONATHAN DECKER, LMFT;
& W. JARED DUPREE, PHD, MBA

"PUT YOUR EAR DOWN CLOSE TO YOUR SOUL AND LISTEN HARD."[1]
—ANNE SEXTON

PATRICK R. STEFFEN, PhD, *has conducted research in the areas of clinical health psychology, stress reduction, and biofeedback, with specific interests in culture, spirituality, and health. He is particularly interested in the Hispanic Paradox and how disadvantaged groups display resiliency and positive adaptation in spite of significant stressors. He is on the editorial boards for the journals* Annals of Behavioral Medicine, Journal of Behavioral Medicine, *and* Frontiers in Psychology, *and he is on the board of directors for the Association for Applied Psychophysiology and Biofeedback. He has authored and coauthored articles in* Psychosomatic Medicine, Annals of Behavioral Medicine, Journal of Behavioral Medicine, American Journal of Hypertension, Ethnicity and Disease, Mindfulness, *and* Mental Health, Religion, and Culture; *and he has also coauthored chapters in the* Oxford Handbook of Health Psychology *and the* Handbook of Primary Care Psychology. *Dr. Steffen is a professor of psychology at Brigham Young University and is the director of the doctoral program in clinical psychology. Before coming to BYU, Dr. Steffen was a postdoctoral research fellow in cardiovascular behavioral medicine at Duke University Medical Center. He received his PhD and master's degrees at the University of Miami in clinical health psychology and a bachelor's degree in psychology with minors in statistics and philosophy from Brigham Young University.*

JONATHAN DECKER, MS, *is a licensed marriage and family therapist specializing in couples therapy, blended families, singles' guidance, bereavement, and working with adolescents. He holds a master's degree in marriage and family therapy from Auburn University and a bachelor's in clinical psychology from Brigham Young University. Jonathan is the clinic manager of the Online Center for Couples and Families (NetFamilyTherapy.com), which offers online webcam sessions to clientele in various states. He is a certified facilitator of the singles' class "How to Avoid Falling in Love with a Jerk or Jerkette." He also reviews Hollywood films from a parent's perspective at www.MovieDad.com. He is married with four children.*

INTRODUCTION

Viktor Frankl (1905–1997) was a practicing neurologist and psychiatrist when World War II began. Because he was a Jew, he was taken prisoner by the Nazis in 1942 and sent to live in concentration camps, where most of his family died. He details his horrific experiences in the book *Man's Search for Meaning*. In spite of the unimaginable hardships he faced, he is remembered today as a man whose life exemplified meaning and purpose.

Frankl frequently repeated two beliefs that he said helped him endure the horrible suffering of the Holocaust. He wrote, first, "suffering ceases to be suffering when it finds a meaning." And second, "he who has a strong enough why can endure almost any how." He believed that life has meaning under all circumstances, even the most miserable and difficult situations. The ultimate freedom, Frankl taught, was the freedom to choose our own thoughts and attitudes, something that the Nazis could not take away from him. The greatest truth or meaning that Frankl found was that love is the highest goal to which people can aspire, that "the salvation of man is through love and in love."[2]

In many respects, the life of Viktor Frankl is a paradox. Abraham Maslow, a famous humanistic psychologist, developed an influential theory of needs stating that self-actualization comes only after meeting more basic needs such as food, safety, and social connection. Viktor Frankl's example, however, turns this all upside down. Dr. Frankl did not have adequate food, safety, or social connection. And yet he is the epitome of self-actualization. In spite of the horror of his surroundings, he found deeper meaning in serving and helping others and working for a better future. In fact, Frankl argued that instead of striving for self-actualization, we should strive for self-transcendence.

Frankl stated the following:

> Being human always points, and is directed, to something, to someone, other than oneself—be it a meaning to fulfill or another human being to encounter. The more one forgets himself by giving himself to a cause to serve or another person to love, the more human he is and the more he actualizes himself. What is called self-actualization is not an attainable aim at all, for the simple reason that the more one would strive for it, the more he would miss it. In other words, self-actualization is possible only as a side-effect of self-transcendence.[3]

Frankl taught that we are made up of mind, body, and spirit that are interdependent, with the spirit being key. It is spirit that allows wholeness, enables us to exercise our will to meaning, move beyond basic instincts, and achieve our goals. This is the essence of spirituality.

Spirituality involves a search for ultimate truth, a search for meaning in life, experiences with the transcendent, and personal transformation.[4] Whereas religiosity usually involves participation in public worship services, focus on transcendent issues, and membership in a specific religious denomination, spirituality usually involves personal strivings for transcendent meaning and truth. Most people describe themselves as being spiritual at some level even though religious activity has been decreasing in recent years. In fact, the number of people who describe themselves as spiritual but not religious is on the rise.

WHY IS SPIRITUALITY GOOD FOR YOUR PHYSICAL HEALTH?

Aaron Antonovsky, a researcher who studied Holocaust survivors in Israel in the 1960s and 1970s, noted that almost one-third of survivors were in excellent mental and physical health in spite of having gone through one of the most horrific episodes in the history of the world.[5] He was actually shocked that so many were doing so well. It is interesting to note that after the Holocaust, Viktor Frankl went on to live a robust life and died at the age of ninety-two. In order to understand what contributed to these miraculous health outcomes, Antonovsky conducted a series of studies to see what set these people apart. In study after study, he found three factors that stood out: meaning, comprehensibility, and manageability. Those that thrived in spite of adversity had a deep sense of meaning and purpose in life. They had strong reasons to continue pressing forward, even when things looked hopeless. These individuals were able to make sense of life stressors (comprehensibility) in a way that helped them cope effectively. And these individuals actively worked (manageability) to overcome obstacles and move forward.

Antonovsky's research findings on the importance of life meaning have been replicated across numerous studies. People who seek and strive for deeper meaning in life do better both mentally and physically than those who focus on hedonistic or materialistic pleasures.[6] These two approaches to life (meaning-focused versus pleasure-focused) are also called the *eudaimonic* and *hedonic* perspectives. Psychology has typically focused on the hedonic perspective, assuming that people are mostly motivated to increase pleasure and reduce pain. Recent research, however, has found that the eudaimonic perspective, or meaning-based perspective, is related to better health. Interestingly, people would rather live a meaningful life that is difficult than an easy life that is empty of meaning.

The eudaimonic perspective focuses on meaning, growth, and positive relationships with others as key motivations in life. Pleasure motivation is not considered bad; rather, pleasure is a result of living a life that is focused on meaning, growth, and positive relationships. Measures of eudaimonic and hedonistic perspectives are correlated, and if a person is living eudaimonically, then they will necessarily experience hedonic joy as well. Striving to satisfy eudaimonic desires typically leads to hedonistic pleasure, but striving for hedonistic pleasures does not necessarily satisfy eudaimonic desires. For example, some activities might momentarily produce pleasure but do not produce wellness. Taking mind-altering drugs can produce short-term pleasure, but in the long-term lead to addiction and suffering. Therefore, in the eudaimonic perspective subjective, pleasure is not the same thing as well-being.

In addition to a deeper sense of meaning in life, spirituality contributes to physical health through increased healthy behaviors and goals and better self-control. Spiritual individuals are more likely to view their bodies as sacred and something to be cared for and nurtured. Accordingly, spiritual individuals are less likely to use tobacco, excessive alcohol, or illicit drugs. They are more likely to engage in physical activity and exercise and engage in health-care practices such as regular doctor visits. They also set healthy goals for themselves, and over time are more likely to increase physical activity and decrease tobacco use. Finally, spiritual individuals are able to delay gratification and exert more self-control in their health behaviors. People with good self-control report better mood and decreased anger, have healthier personality characteristics (more agreeable, conscientious, and emotionally stable), and have better social relationships. This is also related to meaning in life, with higher meaning in life being related to better self-control and delay of gratification. This is likely because if you have a strong enough reason for doing something, you will be able to exert self-control.

Spirituality also contributes to positive health outcomes through decreased responsiveness to life stressors. Stress can have a huge impact on physical health, and anything that helps us cope better with stress is going to have a positive effect on our health. Individuals with a higher sense of meaning in life report experiencing less negative stress and live longer than those whose lives seem devoid of meaning. In terms of life suffering, believing that there can be meaning in suffering increases our ability to cope effectively and reduces our physiological stress response during these difficult times. Specifically, spiritual individuals have lower blood pressure, decreased inflammation, and lower fasting glucose levels,[7] and increased parasympathetic and cardiac control during stress.[8]

SPIRITUALITY AND OVERCOMING ADVERSITY

A growing body of research indicates that many people are able to turn adversity and trauma into positive growth experiences. The work of has found that positive change often occurs as a result of struggling with highly difficult life experiences.[9] In John 16:33, Christ said, "In the world ye shall have tribulation: but be of good cheer; I have overcome the world." People experiencing adversity and trauma frequently report stronger relationships with others, more meaning in life, and increased spirituality after the trauma. This line of research is related to the eudaimonic perspective. Whereas in the hedonic perspective adversity is something to be avoided, in the eudaimonic perspective adversity is embraced as a challenge and provides meaning to life.

When I [Dr. DuPree] was working in Mississisppi, I remember working with a number of young men that had experienced extreme amounts of adversity. Experiencing abandonment and abuse from their parents, they had been homeless and witnessed horrors at a young age as they were passed from foster care to relatives to the streets, off and on. In my mind, I called them the "forgotten boys" because no one seemed to care. I learned a lot from them as I got to know them. Although they were still trying to heal, their spirituality embraced life. They did not blame or seek revenge; they wanted to help others and let go of the pain by loving others. They felt it was their spiritual mission to make sure the same thing didn't happen to others. Their spiritual understanding was helping them break a cycle of abuse, addiction, and pain.

Minorities and lower-income individuals typically have worse health outcomes relative to whites and higher-income individuals. However, minorities and lower-income people who exhibit higher levels of spirituality do not show a health disadvantage.[10] Even though they still show less hedonistic well-being (score lower on measures of happiness), they show higher levels of eudaimonic well-being (score higher on measures of meaning and strong social bonds) and better health outcomes. Spiritual people with less income and education appear to derive greater benefit from spirituality than those higher in income and education. People with high materialistic motivations, on the other hand, that have less income and education have negative health outcomes.

Spirituality appears to play a significant role in the Hispanic Paradox.[11] The Hispanic Paradox is the fact that Hispanic immigrants have significantly less income and education relative to non-Hispanic blacks and whites, and yet they can have better health outcomes. Many immigrants describe their reasons for immigration and the process of immigration in spiritual tones and attribute their success in life transition to God. As a group, Mexican immigrants in particular tend to be one of the most religious groups in the United

States, with one study finding that Mexican immigrants were the most religious of any group in the United States.[12] In spite of having significantly lower income and less education than whites, Mexican immigrants have lower incidence of diseases such as cardiovascular disease and live longer than whites.[13]

MARRIAGE AND SPIRITUALITY

Spirituality is a key component of a successful, happy marriage. As mentioned previously, Maslow proposed that self-actualization occurs after the meeting of basic needs. Yet those who see marriage as a means to get their own needs met (social, sexual, self-image, or otherwise) are often disappointed. They tend to complain that they aren't "getting what they need" out of the relationship and that they expect more from their partner. However, those who see marriage as an opportunity for self-*transcendence* (through serving, comforting, and helping their spouse) tend to achieve self-actualization as a by-product.

Spiritual love is an act of giving, while selfish love is an act of taking. The latter seeks personal hedonic gratification, while the former transcends natural selfishness to find meaning in lightening the burdens of another, in true eudaimonic fashion. A noted theologian and author explained that "happiness in marriage is not so much a matter of romance as it is an anxious concern for the comfort and well-being of one's companion."[14] Of course, one's partner must reciprocate to some degree. One-sided service and love often leads to one partner feeling entitled and the other feeling used. But if both partners prioritize the other's wants and needs, finding meaning in caring for one another, these are the makings of a successful marriage. For example, I [Dr. DuPree] have worked with many couples that make a shift from selfish love to spiritual love when they let go of fear. They are afraid that their spouse doesn't love them, so they become concerned with all the things their spouse is or isn't doing that "proves" they don't love them (not making the bed, not helping with the kids, not engaging in intimacy, not giving a compliment, and so on). Spiritual love is built on faith and concern for the other's well-being. Rather than worrying about what the other spouse is not doing, there is a desire to understand him or her, become well-acquainted with his or her wants and needs, and seek to meet those wants and needs. Thus, John helps Lisa with the dishes, knowing they are both tired from the day. Theresa gives Justin a compliment and thanks him for being a great husband, not expecting anything in return. Sarah and Brad make an effort to talk to one another about their day because they want to be a part of each other's lives.

Even with regards to sex, a spiritually-grounded marriage achieves pleasure as a by-product, not as an end in and of itself. In his book *How to Avoid Falling in Love with a Jerk,* Dr. John Vann Epp explains that the key to great sex is a couples' growth in a meaningful relationship. His review of the research shows that married couples are more likely to report being sexually satisfied than singles or cohabitators. This may be because sex in a healthy marriage is particularly meaningful as the culmination of emotional, intellectual, and spiritual intimacy. Dr. Van Epp explains that getting to know someone on a profound level, being able to trust them, rely on them, and commit to them fully creates a level of comfort and security that maximizes sexual connection and meaning.[15]

Steffen notes that spirituality involves, among other things, personal transformation. While marital strain may occur if partners expect too much change from one another, it is perfectly natural in a healthy marriage for spouses to "bring out the best" in each other.[16] Through the transformative, spiritual influence of marital union, partners learn from one another. They change how they interact in order to foster harmony. The spiritual results of a happy union include increased patience, self-sacrifice, accountability, and kindness.

Van Epp reviewed existing research on spirituality and marriage, finding that couples with a high level of compatibility with regard to spiritual values are more likely to have successful relationships.[17] In couples where spirituality is intertwined with religion, sharing the same faith statistically leads to a higher rate of marital satisfaction and endurance. However, couples of different faiths can be happily (and lastingly) married if they share the spiritual value of respecting one another's beliefs, finding common ground, and not pressuring each other to change. Couples who have shared spiritual values of nurturing growth and prioritizing their relationship, as well as shared views on whether to have, and how to raise, children, have a higher likelihood of a building a lasting, healthy relationship than those who do not.

SPIRITUALITY AND PSYCHOTHERAPY

People generally seek psychotherapy with the aim of alleviating pain of some kind. Counselors help their clients overcome suffering and achieve well-being through the eudaimonic quest for meaning, growth, and healthy personal relationships. With regards to meaning (to paraphrase Frankl), purpose helps clients to endure their sorrows, while meaninglessness makes these unbearable. It therefore behooves the therapist to assist their client in finding a why for their pain.

One thing Frankl found was that everything people suffer empowers them to help others. If they let it, pain can make them more compassionate, wiser, and able to empathize. Clients often feel that those best qualified to help them are those who have passed through similar ordeals. They gravitate toward therapists who have "been there." They expect the clinician to be able to relate and to give good advice on how to get through their problems.

Of course, it isn't necessary for therapists to have endured similar situations in order to help. They can sympathize and call upon their education to help the client see that one "reason" for their suffering is to empower him or her (the client) to commiserate with others, to ease pain, and to assure others that they're not alone. If clients suffer because of poor choices, therapists guide them to help others avoid making the same mistakes. Clients discover the truth spoken by Gandhi: "The best way to find yourself is to lose yourself in the service of others."[18] The client gains an empowering new identity, not as a sufferer but as a comforter and an inspiration to others.

In facilitating a client's search for meaning, clinicians encounter less resistance from clients if they work *within* the framework of the client's existing spiritual (and religious) beliefs, instead of challenging and negating them. In his book *Staring at the Sun: Overcoming the Terror of Death*, esteemed psychotherapist Irvin D. Yalom argues that, even if a clinician personally disagrees with a client's spiritual or religious beliefs, he or she should not challenge these deeply held worldviews, especially if they are a source of strength, comfort, and meaning to the client.[19]

I [Dr. DuPree] remember working with a young woman back East who was questioning some beliefs that were deeply held family traditions. She was also having difficulty seeing "eye to eye" with her father on many issues in her life. Her father was a religious leader in their faith, and there was pressure to not embarrass the family. As I worked with her, she used some of these disagreements as a time to truly explore who she is as a woman, daughter, fiancée, and human being. We decided together that there was no need to make any hard decisions about any beliefs at this time; rather, she could use this time to explore her life in general. Letting her father know that she was in an "exploratory" mode gave them permission to have some great conversations together and get to know each other more. Equally, as she became more aware of who she is as a person, she allowed others to get to know her more. Her relationships with her father, family, and God were strengthened. We never discussed the correctness of a certain belief during our time. We discussed the way in which beliefs are formed and discovered and changed over time. Complete freedom was given to find them for herself. A good psychotherapist will guide and facilitate a process of personal discovery.

SPIRITUAL PRACTICES

There are many practices that are designed to increase spirituality, and most religious and philosophical traditions have spiritual practices built into the belief system. Huston Smith, the famous professor of comparative religion, argued, "The empowering theological and metaphysical truths of the worlds religions are inspired. When religions are sifted for those truths . . . they look like the data banks that house the winnowed wisdom of the human race."[20] Key spiritual practices distilled from these wisdom traditions include prayer, meditation, study and contemplation of sacred texts, and giving service to others.

Prayer

This is an incredibly common spiritual practice, with almost 75 percent of Americans reporting that they pray at least weekly and 57 percent praying at least daily.[21] *Prayer*, from the Latin "to seek earnestly or entreat," involves sincere supplication to attain communion with God or a higher power. The LDS Bible Dictionary defines prayer as "the act by which the will of the Father and will of the child are brought into correspondence with each other. Prayer is a form of work, and is an appointed means for obtaining the highest of all blessings."[22] Through prayer, people contemplate and reflect on life meaning and their relationship to a higher or transcendent power and work to achieve connection with that power. Frequent prayer is related to decreased stress, increased meaning and life, and improved health.[23] Prayer is also a common feature of public worship services and helps a group or community grow stronger and grow closer together through shared intention. If you have never prayed, various faiths and belief systems suggest different methods. In general, we recommend viewing prayer as communication between you and a higher power. In simple terms, begin to speak or communicate to a higher power in your mind, on paper, or out loud. Take time to listen to your thoughts, intuitions, emotions, and spiritual experiences as you seek to listen to your higher power.

Meditation

Meditation is also a common spiritual practice and is similar to prayer in that it often involves contemplation and reflection. The practice of meditation and prayer is often integrated and the one can help deepen the other. LDS president David O. McKay taught that we do not take sufficient time to meditate. He said, "Meditation is the language of the soul. It is defined as 'a form of private devotion or spiritual exercise, consisting in deep, continued reflection on some religious theme.' Meditation is a form of prayer."[24] He explained that we can come closer to the Lord than we imagine when we learn to meditate— that meditation provides an excellent opportunity for our spirits to be taught by the Spirit. Given that prayer is a form of work, meditation can increase ability to engage in that work.

Meditation leads to a number of positive mental and physical health outcomes. Those who meditate regularly have reduced stress, depression, and anxiety, as well as lower blood pressure and improved immune function.[25] An additional benefit of meditative practice is increased awareness and attention, which is critical for learning.[26] Although meditation may appear difficult or even impossible to practice, anyone can develop awareness. Development of meditation ability is gradual and requires regular practice.

Similar to prayer, if you have never engaged in meditation, it may be easier to view meditation as purposeful thinking. In other words, find a quiet place in which you can spend some time thinking about a particular topic. Some people meditate for relaxation, while others meditate for clarity or focus. You may want to think about all the simple joys in your life, like people, experiences, blessings, and nature. You could meditate about a particular area in your life, like a certain hobby or passion. You could set goals or meditate on a vision for a new project or on particular challenge in your life. Part of meditation involves allowing yourself to have time to think about that topic and not allow distractions to get in the way. Thus, it would be important to set aside a specific amount of time, a specific purpose to the meditation, and a specific place that allows you to engage in meditation.

Mindfulness Meditation

This is a particularly popular form of meditation, as discussed in chapter 6. In mindfulness meditation, the focus is on being in the moment with nonjudgmental awareness. We are often unaware of our moment-to-moment experience, and practicing mindfulness helps us to be centered in the present moment. Much of mental suffering stems from rumination, fears, and negative self-evaluations that are not usually present-focused. We ruminate about the past or worry about the future but do not live in the present. Learning to be in the present moment and acknowledge life as it is helps us to rise out of negative thinking.

A common misconception of mindfulness practice is that accepting things as they are is the same as giving up and not trying to achieve life goals. If you imagine your journey in life as being represented on a map, then acceptance is being aware of where you are exactly on that map. In order to move toward valued goals, you first need to recognize where you are starting. When our mental focus is rumination and worry, we are avoiding being in the present moment, and we become stuck because we do not recognize where we are or what desired paths we would like to follow.

When we engage in mindful meditation, the focus is on the here and now. Similar to regular meditation, you want to find a specific place and time that fits your needs. The topic of the meditation will be the here and now, with special attention to all of your senses. Feel the breeze and the warmth of the sun, listen to the sounds around you, pay attention to how your body is responding (heartbeat, skin, muscles, and so on), and allow yourself to live in the moment.

Studying Sacred Texts or Scriptures

Personal study is a powerful way to grow spiritually. In order to fully engage in spiritual practices such as prayer and meditation, we must first learn about and understand these practices. As Huston Smith noted, religious teachings and practices represent the stored wisdom of the human race. This wisdom is stored in sacred texts and scriptures, and regular study of these texts helps us to grow spiritually and learn spiritual truths that can be applied in our daily lives. Scripture study is associated with better mental and physical health.[27, 28, 29]

One spiritual truth that is found in all major sacred texts is serving others,[30] with serving others viewed as a core aspect of spirituality. For example, throughout the New Testament, service to others is taught and exemplified. Christ washed the feet of His disciples and taught them, "A new commandment I give unto you, That ye love one another; as I have loved you, that ye also love one another" (John 13:34). Modern research finds that giving service is related to better mental and physical health. Volunteering time and effort leads to better mental health outcomes and greater longevity.[31, 32, 33] Apparently in contradiction to many modern beliefs, one study found that giving social support predicted better health outcomes than receiving social support, or as the Apostle Paul said, "It is more blessed to give than to receive" (Acts 20:35). In short, people who serve others live longer, healthier, happier lives.

CONCLUSION

Spirituality plays a key role in mental and physical health. Spiritual individuals are better able to cope with stress and deal with traumatic events, have lower levels of depression and anxiety, and healthier cardiovascular and immune function. Probably because of this, spiritual individuals live longer than others. The life of Viktor Frankl provides an excellent example of how spirituality impacts health. In spite of the horrors he experienced during the Holocaust, he was able to live a deeply meaningful life and make a significant impact on the world. He taught the paradoxical truth that only through self-transcendence (serving and loving others) can we grow and become self-actualized. The challenge for us in our spiritual growth is to transcend our self-focus. We can all grow spiritually by seeking self-transcendence through prayer, meditation, study of sacred texts, and giving loving service to others.

NOTES

1. Anne Sexton, as quoted on "Anne Sexton," The Poetry Foundation, accessed October 16, 2015, http://www.poetryarchive.org/poet/anne-sexton.

2. V. Frankl, *Man's Search for Meaning* (Boston, MA: Washington Square Press).

3. Ibid., 133.

4. P. R. Steffen, "Approaching religiosity/spirituality and health from the eudaimonic perspective," *Social and Personality Psychology Compass* 6 (2012): 70–82.

5. A. Antonovsky, "The Salutogenic Perspective: Toward a new view of health and illness," *Advances* 4 (1987): 47–55.

6. P. R. Steffen, "Approaching religiosity/spirituality and health from the eudaimonic perspective."

7. J. Holt-Lunstad et al., "Understanding the connection between spiritual well-being and physical health: An examination of ambulatory blood pressure, inflammation, blood lipids, and fasting glucose," *Journal of Behavioral Medicine* 34 (2011): 477–88.

8. G. G. Berntson et al., "Spirituality and autonomic cardiac control," *Annals of Behavioral Medicine* 35 (2008): 198–208.

9. R. G. Tedeschi and L. G. Calhoun, "Posttraumatic growth: Conceptual foundations and empirical evidence," *Psychological Inquiry* 15 (2004): 1–18.

10. P. R. Steffen et al., "Religious coping, ethnicity, and ambulatory blood pressure," *Psychosomatic Medicine* 63 (2001): 523–30.

11. J. M. Ruiz and P. R. Steffen, "Latino Health" (2011) in H.S. Friedman, ed. *The Oxford Handbook of Health Psychology* (New York: Oxford University Press), 805–23.

12. L. Hao and R. W. Johnson, "Economic, cultural, and social origins of emotional well-being: Comparisons of immigrants and natives at midlife," *Research on Aging* 22 (2000): 599–629.

13. J. M. Ruiz, P. R. Steffen, and T. B. Smith, "The Hispanic Mortality Paradox: A systematic review and meta-analysis of the longitudinal literature," *American Journal of Public Health* (2013): 103, e52-e60, doi:10.2105/AJPH. 2012.301103.

14. G. B. Hinckley, "What God Hath Joined Together," *Ensign*, May 1991.

15. J. Van Epp, *How to Avoid Falling in Love with a Jerk* (New York, NY: McGraw-Hill, 2008).

16. P. R. Steffen, "Approaching religiosity/spirituality and health from the eudaimonic perspective."

17. J. Van Epp, *How to Avoid Falling in Love with a Jerk*.

18. Mohandas Karamchand Gandhi, as quoted in "12 Great Quotes From Gandhi On His Birthday," October 2, 2012, http://www.forbes.com/sites/ashoka/2012/10/02/12-great-quotes-from-gandhi-on-his-birthday/.

19. I. D. Yalom, *Staring at the Sun: Overcoming the Terror of Death* (San Francisco, CA: Jossey-Bass Publishing, 2009).

20. H. Smith, *The World's Religions* (San Francisco, CA: Harper, 1991), 5.

21. General Social Survey, 2010.

22. LDS Bible Dictionary, s.v. "Prayer."

23. C. A. Lewis, M. J. Breslin, and S. Dein, "Prayer and mental health: An introduction to this special issue of mental health, religion & culture," *Mental Health, Religion, & Culture* 11 (2008): 1–7.

24. D. O. McKay, in Conference Report, April 1967, or "Consciousness of God: Supreme goal of life," *Ensign*, May 1967, 84–8.

25. P. Grossman, L. Niemann, S. Schmidt, and H. Walach, "Mindfulness-based stress reduction and health benefits: a meta-analysis," *Journal of Psychosomatic Research* 57 (2004): 35–43.

26. J. T. Ramsburg and R. J. Youmans, "Meditation in the higher education classroom: mediation training improves student knowledge retention during lectures," *Mindfulness* 5 (2014): 431–41.

27. Y. Chida, A. Steptoe, and L. H. Powell, "Religiosity/spirituality and mortality," *Psychotherapy and Psychosomatics*, 78 (2009): 81–90.

28. M. E. McCullough et al., "Religious involvement and mortality: A meta-analytic review," *Health Psychology* 19 (2000): 211–22.

29. L. H. Powell, L. Shahabi, and C. E. Thoresen, "Religion and spirituality: Linkages to physical health," *American Psychologist* 58 (2003): 36–52.

30. H. Smith, *The World's Religions*, 5.

31. P. L. Dulin and R. D. Hill, "Relationships between altruistic activity and positive and negative affect among low-income older adult service providers," *Aging and Mental Health* 7 (2003): 294–99.

32. D. Oman, C. E. Thoresen, and K. McMahon, "Volunteerism and mortality among the community dwelling elderly," *Journal of Health Psychology* 4 (1999): 301–16.

33. C. Schwartz et al., "Altruistic social interest behaviors are associated with better mental health," *Psychosomatic Medicine* 65 (2003): 778–85.

SECTI⚙N
5

FINDING LIFE BALANCE

"To every thing there is a season, and a time to every purpose under the heaven: A time to be born, and a time to die; a time to plant, and a time to pluck up that which is planted; A time to kill, and a time to heal; a time to break down, and a time to build up; A time to weep, and a time to laugh; a time to mourn, and a time to dance; A time to cast away stones, and a time to gather stones together; a time to embrace, and a time to refrain from embracing; A time to get, and a time to lose; a time to keep, and a time to cast away; A time to rend, and a time to sew; a time to keep silence, and a time to speak; A time to love, and a time to hate; a time of war, and a time of peace."

—Ecclesiastes 3:1–8

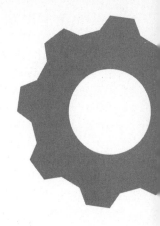

15 STRESS AND HEALTH

BY PATRICK R. STEFFEN, PHD

"GIVE YOUR STRESS WINGS AND LET IT FLY."[1]
—TERRI GUILLEMETS

Editor's note: If you are one who struggles with stress, this chapter is a message of hope. If you, like me, are prone to taking on too much or allowing worries and deadlines to impact your health, please read on. The research Dr. Steffen shares in this chapter will help you reinvent the role of stress in your life. I hope you will have the same experience I had as I learned that stress is only a negative force in our lives if we perceive it to be negative. Understanding how to use stress as a tool will leave you feeling more empowered, confident, and at peace.

INTRODUCTION

Charles and Thomas were two midlevel managers who lost their jobs due to company downsizing. Charles was understandably distressed by the situation and worried about how this would affect his family and future. He used this energy to seek diligently for a new job. Although this process took much longer than he would have liked, he eventually found a suitable position. Thomas was also understandably distressed by the situation and worried about how this would affect his family and future. He became depressed and anxious about his ability to find a similar good paying job and developed difficulties sleeping and eating. After several failed attempts in his job search, he stopped searching because everything seemed futile. As time went on, he withdrew from family and friends and become despondent.

Why did Charles and Thomas, who appeared similar on the surface, have such different results in response to a significant life stressor? A recently published research article sheds light on why this can happen. A national study involving over twenty-eight thousand people revealed that stress impacted health only in those that *perceived* that stress negatively impacts health.[2]

Importantly, those that perceived stress as manageable did not have negative outcomes. Stress itself is not bad. Rather, it is the *perception* that stress is bad that is related to physical health problems and early death. Perception is the key.

WHAT IS STRESS?

Stress is the balance between our perceived abilities and our perceived life demands. If we perceive we are capable to meet our life demands, then stress energizes us to work and succeed. If we perceive that our life demands are greater than our abilities to cope, then stress leads to anxiety, depression, and negative physical health outcomes. If we consistently believe that our life demands are greater than our ability to cope over years and decades, then stress will contribute to poor health and increased health risks such as major depression, cardiovascular disease, and immune problems and will likely contribute to an early death.

The first study to experimentally demonstrate the negative effects of stress on health in humans was conducted by Sheldon Cohen and colleagues at Carnegie Mellon University in Pittsburgh, Pennsylvania.[3] Cohen recruited a random sample of participants to stay in a motel for six days, and on the first day had each person exposed to a cold virus. He then measured their stress levels and sampled nasal secretions each day to see who would actually catch a cold. At the end of the six days, he found that those with the highest levels of perceived stress were the most likely to catch a cold. Cohen and colleagues have repeated this experiment in a number of different conditions and found similar results: those more predisposed to negative stress are more likely to get sick.[4]

HOW DOES PSYCHOLOGICAL STRESS LEAD TO DISEASE RISK?

So how does negative psychological stress turn into physical health problems? To answer this question, it is helpful to look at how the body works to establish health and then look at how this can go wrong when people are chronically stressed (see Sapolsky, 2004, for a more thorough review). To survive and thrive, the human body has several built-in survival mechanisms. The most widely known is the fight-or-flight response. When we feel threatened or challenged, the fight-or-flight response kicks in to help us mobilize energy resources and prepare for action. In response to brief stressors, this is a highly adaptive response that helps us to cope well with stress. The goal of this response is to maintain balance or homeostasis, balancing internal needs (digestion, sleep, repair) with external demands (work, deadlines, children, bad drivers, and so on).

However, if the fight-or-flight response is chronically activated over time, it can lead to physical health problems. When life becomes unbalanced with external demands taking more time and energy, there will be less time and energy for basic internal needs such as digestion, sleep, and repair. This leads to a weakened physiological state where we are more prone to illness and disease. Stress does not usually directly cause disease; rather, it leads to physiological dysregulation where disease is more likely to occur. Prolonged physiological dysregulation can lead to problems such as ulcers, hypertension, and decreased immune function.

We do not always respond to stress with the fight-or-flight response. Research studies indicate that we can also respond with what is called the tend-and-befriend response. This response, which is seen more prominently in women, involves seeking and providing social support during times of stress. As humans we are social beings and we benefit greatly from feeling connected to others, receiving help from others, and giving help to others. As the saying goes, there is strength in numbers, and just the perception of feeling supported reduces the physiological stress response. Interestingly, even having a pet dog present during times of stress (such as giving a public speech) reduces the physiological stress response. The tend-and-befriend response also has a third possibility: "defend," which has been shown in mothers of young children, with the mothers showing increased aggression in response to threat to their family. Because "tend and befriend and defend" is socially oriented and builds social bonds, it is an effective way to cope with and reduce stress.

As with tend and befriend and defend, the fight-or-flight response also has three components with the third being "freeze." Therefore, the complete name is "fight or flight or freeze." In most responses to stress, the first response is to freeze and evaluate the situation before acting, which is typically also the case in "tend and befriend and defend," where a time to evaluate is needed before choosing a course of action. Thinking in terms of adaptation and survival, freeze can be a very adaptive response to acute stress. For example, if a white rabbit sitting in the snow sees a predator, the rabbit's first response will be to freeze and see if the predator has seen it. If the predator does not see the rabbit and moves on, then the rabbit does not have to engage in flight and use up a lot of energy. The same is true with humans. The ideal is to first evaluate a situation before committing to a course of action that might be unnecessary and misuse precious resources.

Although freezing in response to an acute stressor is adaptive, engaging in freezing behavior in response to chronic stress is damaging. If we are chronically frozen by worry, anxiety, or fear, we will fail to engage in life and miss out on opportunities for growth and happiness. As with fight and flight, having balance is crucial. We want to respond effectively to life's challenges and take advantage of possibilities that are important to us as they come our way. After pausing and evaluating our situation, we want to act; we want to choose a course of action that lines up with our personal values. If we get stuck in analysis paralysis, where we are always planning and ruminating but not doing, we will not be able to achieve our goals or dreams.

WHAT IS THE PHYSIOLOGICAL STRESS RESPONSE?

There are two key pathways through which the body mobilizes for stress that contribute to the physiological stress response. We will call these the fast-response system and the slow-response system. The fast-response system involves the hormones adrenaline and noradrenaline (also called epinephrine and norepinephrine). The first part of the "fight or flight or freeze" response is the release of adrenaline and noradrenaline into the bloodstream that leads to increases in heart rate and blood pressure. The increased pressure leads to faster blood flow, getting energy to the major muscle groups quickly so the body will be able to engage in fight or flight. Over the history of humankind, this has been a very effective method for dealing with life threats. In today's society, however, fighting and running away are typically not effective solutions to problems. Most of our stressors are social in nature, and it is not appropriate to hit someone or run away screaming (even when we wish we could).

The freeze option is typically what people choose. That is, something stressful happens and the body prepares for action with the release of adrenaline, but no action is taken. Chronic activation of the fast-response system is associated with increased anxiety and increased risk for high blood pressure. We feel worried and we feel tense, and these feelings remain because we do not engage in active coping. If this is our habitual way of responding to life stressors, then we will likely develop an anxiety disorder and cardiovascular problems such as high blood pressure. If, on the other hand, we learn to use the energy of the fight-or-flight response for active coping then we can channel this energy to good purpose. It is interesting that feeling an adrenaline rush and feeling anxiety and fear are both based on adrenaline release in the bloodstream. The main difference is in the perception: do you perceive the stressor as a challenge or as a threat?

The slow-response system involves the release of the hormone cortisol into the bloodstream. Cortisol is primarily a metabolic hormone (involved in energy regulation), which makes it an ideal part of the stress response.

Whereas adrenaline and noradrenaline get the blood moving quickly, cortisol helps in getting energy such as glucose into the bloodstream. The reason that cortisol is part of the slow-response system is that in stressful situations that resolve quickly, an increase in energy might not be needed. Therefore, you have a quick release of adrenaline, but if it does not last long enough there is no need for extra energy to be sent to the muscles.

Cortisol is considered to be a key factor in long-term chronic stress. When we perceive our stressors as continual or fairly constant over the months and years of our lives, then our cortisol levels will increase. Chronically high cortisol levels have at least two main negative effects. First, high cortisol levels are immunosuppressive, making it harder for your immune system to fight off infectious disease. Second, high cortisol levels at bedtime interfere with sleeping well. Disrupted sleep over time can develop into insomnia, which is a key risk factor for the development of major depression. In fact, over 50 percent of individuals with major depression have elevated cortisol levels. Robert Sapolsky, the famous Stanford biologist, argues that chronic stress and major depression is really the same thing (see Sapolsky, 2004). In truth, physiologically it is very difficult to distinguish someone with a chronic stress disorder from someone with major depression. They both show the same alterations in cortisol and brain functioning. Major depression then is really about being overwhelmed and worn down by chronic life stressors.

COPING WITH CHRONIC LIFE STRESSORS

Is it possible to effectively cope with chronic life stressors? Fortunately, the answer is yes. As noted in the previous chapter, perhaps the most famous example of someone coping with horrific chronic stress is Viktor Frankl. Despite witnessing unimaginable atrocities and losing most of his immediate family, Frankl was able to find meaning in his suffering through serving and helping those around him (see Frankl, 1997, for a full account).[5] Now let's consider the research of Aaron Antonovsky in terms of the stress response. Perhaps one of the reasons that such a large number of Antonovsky's research subjects were able to find meaning in their concentration camp experiences had to do with their ability to *perceive* that the stressors they were experiencing were manageable.[6] As noted previously, this healthy group of survivors was noticeably different from the others in regards to the deep sense of meaning they experienced in life.

A well-known result of exposure to severe chronic stress is posttraumatic stress disorder, or PTSD. However, a large number of people exposed to trauma never develop PTSD, and a significant portion experience what is called "posttraumatic growth." Posttraumatic growth is positive change that occurs as a result of struggling with highly difficult life experiences, turning adversity and trauma into positive growth experiences.[7] People experiencing trauma and significant adversity also frequently report increased meaning in life, stronger relationships with others, and increased spirituality. Being able to make sense of difficult life experiences helps people to cope. As Frankl said, "suffering ceases to be suffering when it finds a meaning."[8]

Another concept to consider when coping with chronic stress is called "shift and persist." Growing up in a dangerous inner city neighborhood or in poverty are chronic stressors. The stress of growing up in these environments as a child is directly linked to negative physical and mental health outcomes as an adult. Researchers Edith Chen and Greg Miller have noted that children in these environments are able to cope well with chronic stress by learning to "shift and persist."[9] That is, they learn to shift themselves by learning to accept stress for what it is and adapting by reappraising the meaning of stress, and they persist by holding on to meaning and optimism. A key to this process is children having good role models or mentors who teach them to trust and build good relationships with others, manage their emotions, and build hope for the future.

MOTIVATION TO COPE WITH CHRONIC STRESSORS: HEART DISEASE AND IMMUNE DYSFUNCTION

Why should we do something right now to learn to better cope with chronic stress? The basic answer is we are going to have a lower quality of life and will die sooner than we should if we do not. Chronic stress plays a key role in the development of heart disease and immune dysfunction. Heart disease is the leading cause of death in all Western countries and is primarily the result of lifestyle behaviors (lack of physical activity, poor diet, smoking) and chronic stress. Because the quality and length of our lives is directly related to our lifestyle choices and stress, we can directly make positive changes to our health and longevity by improving how we cope with stress. These changes need to be integrated into everyday life; we can't exercise only on Saturdays and think we have it covered. Developing healthy daily habits are key to coping with stress.

HOW CAN WE COPE BETTER WITH OUR LIFE STRESSORS?

There are four keys to improving how we cope with life. First, we need to identify what is most important and meaningful to us in our lives by clearly defining our values. Time is limited, and we cannot do every good thing that is possible; we need to focus our time on what matters most. Stress management really begins with time management based on clear life values. Second, we need to learn to accept things we cannot change (other people, the weather, and so on) and commit to work on things we can change. Third, we need to make sure we are getting adequate sleep, exercise, and healthy food. These are the building blocks for having a healthy body. And fourth, we need to structure time for rest and recreation in our daily schedules so we do not burn ourselves out. The most successful people in the world do not work nonstop; they have a healthy work-life balance and take time to relax and enjoy life.

1. Values

A helpful way to get clarity about your life values is to imagine your funeral. This might sound morbid, but it is a useful exercise. Imagine that you are attending your funeral in spirit form and listening to what people are saying about you. Think about what you would like them to say about you. What kind of life did you lead? What kind of person were you? What stands out most in people's minds? When conducting these types of thought experiments, people rarely say that they wished they had spent more time at the office or had worked an extra ten hours per week. Rather, people emphasize spending more time with family and friends, serving in the community, and pursuing personally meaningful activities. The important point here is that we clearly identify what is most meaningful to us and build our lives around our most important values.

Perhaps surprisingly, pursuing what we deeply value leads us to not only live a richer and more meaningful life, but it also leads us to be more successful in all areas of life. Researchers Ed Deci and Robert Ryan have conducted literally hundreds of research studies indicating that living according to intrinsically meaningful choices (serving others, personal growth, and so on) leads to enhanced well-being and success, whereas living according to extrinsically orientated motivations (money, fame, and so forth) leads to decreased well-being.[10] When we live our lives according to personally meaningful values, we are energized to be successful in all areas of life, including work.

2. Acceptance and Commitment

It is important to recognize that stress is a normal part of life and is not going to go away.[11] Accepting that life is stressful does not mean that we are giving in or giving up. Acceptance means recognizing the reality of things as they stand and even welcoming the challenges of life. Christ stated in John 16:33, "These things I have spoken unto you, that in me ye might have peace. In the world ye shall have tribulation: but be of good cheer; I have overcome the world." M. Scott Peck, the famous psychotherapist, said, "Life is difficult. This is a great truth, one of the greatest truths. It is a great truth because once we truly see this truth, we transcend it. Once we truly know that life is difficult—once we truly understand and accept it—then life is no longer difficult. Because once it is accepted, the fact that life is difficult no longer matters."[12] We can transform the stressors in our lives by changing our mind-set about the meaning of those stressors.[13]

When we accept the stress of life as a challenge and not as a threat, we can more fully commit to ourselves to live according to our values.[14] When we perceive stress as a threat, we tend to avoid and disengage, which prevents us from taking effective action. Seeing stress as a challenge invigorates us and energizes us to accomplish valued goals. We can commit to live a full and meaningful life *with* our current stressors. We don't have to wait for our stressors to disappear before we begin to live fully. We can immediately work toward valued goals and work to make the world a better place for our families, friends, and communities right now.

3. Lifestyle

To cope effectively with stress, we need a healthy body. The health of our body is a direct function of our daily lifestyle, and a healthy lifestyle consists of adequate sleep, exercise, and healthy food. In a real sense, sleep, exercise, and food are important in medical treatment and can be considered medicine. Many hospitals have sleep medicine clinics, and researchers are now arguing that doctors should prescribe exercise as medicine. The goal of medicine is to maintain health through the prevention, alleviation, and curing of disease. Research shows that sleep, exercise, and diet are all vitally important in disease prevention, and they are also key components in many rehabilitation programs such as cardiac and stroke rehabilitation. In addition to improving physical health, exercise improves mental health and is as effective as antidepressants in alleviating depressive symptoms.[15] Similarly, improved sleep quality is related to improved mood and decreased anxiety as well as improved physical health.

4. Rest and Recreation

Rest and recreation are essential for stress reduction and healthy living. Some people believe that success can only be obtained by working hard and then working harder. Research on highly successful performers has found that rest periods are just as important as practice periods. In a study on expert violinists, it was found that they rarely practice more than ninety minutes at a time before taking at least a twenty-minute break, and they usually only have three practice sessions a day.[16] In fact, research demonstrates that practicing when tired leads to the development of bad skills and habits because the performer does not have sufficient energy to focus effectively on learning the task at hand. Taking time for recreation and hobbies also rejuvenates and strengthens body and mind. The human body appears to be designed for variety, and prolonged focus on one task dulls the mind and reduces performance. Balancing work with rest and recreation improves performance and increases focus.

CONCLUSION

Stress is a part of life that is not going to disappear. The difference between those who are able to manage their lives and be successful and those who are unable is in how stress is perceived. When we perceive stress as a challenge and commit to valued action, then our stress will energize us to engage effectively in life. When we perceive stress as a threat, then we tend to disengage and avoid life's difficulties, which over time will have significant negative effects on our mental and physical health. The good news is that we all can learn to better cope with our life stressors and change how we perceive stress.

An important key to effective coping is identifying what we value most in life and organizing our time and energy around our personal values. We don't have the time to say yes to everything; we need focus our time on what is truly important. With that being said, a key value that everyone benefits from is making time for family, friends, and social connection. When looking back on life, most people wish they had spent more time with loved ones and not more time in the office. Other keys to effective coping include learning to accept what cannot be changed and committing to change what is within our power; keeping our bodies healthy using the prescription of exercise, sleep, and healthy diet; and taking time for regular rest and recreation. By changing how we cope with and perceive stressors in our lives, we will change our health and well-being for the better.

RECOMMENDED READING

- *Why Zebras Don't Get Ulcers*, 3rd Edition, by R. M. Sapolsky (New York: Holt, 2004).

- *Stress, Health & Well-Being: Thriving in the 21st Century* by R. Harrington. (Belmont, CA: Wadsworth, 2013).

NOTES

1. Terri Guillemets, as quoted in Elizabeth J. Tucker *Simply Stress* (Shepherd Creative Learning, 2014).

2. A. Keller, K. Litzelman, L. E. Wisk, T. Maddox, E. R. Cheng, P. D. Creswell, and W. P. Witt, "Does the perception that stress affects health matter? The association with health and mortality," *Health Psychology* 31 (2012): 677–84.

3. S. Cohen, D. A. Tyrell, and A. P. Smith, "Psychological stress and susceptibility to the common cold," *New England Journal of Medicine* 325 (1991): 606–12.

4. S. Cohen, "Keynote presentation at the Eighth International Congress of Behavioral Medicine: The Pittsburgh Common Cold Studies: Psychosocial predictors of susceptibility to respiratory infectious illness," *International Journal of Behavioral Medicine* 12 (2005): 123–31.

5. V. Frankl, *Man's Search for Meaning* (Boston, MA: Washington Square Press).

6. A. Antonovsky, "The Salutogenic Perspective: Toward a new view of health and illness," *Advances* 4 (1987): 47–55.

7. R. G. Tedeschi and L. G. Calhoun, "Posttraumatic growth: Conceptual foundations and empirical evidence," *Psychological Inquiry* 15 (2004): 1–18.

8. Frankl, *Man's Search for Meaning*.

9. E. Chen and G. E. Miller, "'Shift-and-Persist' Strategies: Why low socioeconomic status isn't always bad for health," *Perspectives on Psychological Science* 7 (2012): 135–58.

10. R. M. Ryan and E. L. Deci, "Self-Determination Theory and the facilitation of intrinsic motivation, social development, and well-being," *American Psychologist* 55 (2000): 68–78.

11. S. C. Hayes and S. Smith, *Get out of Your Mind and into Your Life* (Oakland, CA: New Harbinger Publications, Inc., 2005).

12. M. S. Peck, *The Road Less Traveled* (New York: Touchstone, 1978).

13. A. J. Crum, P. Salovey, and S. Achor, "Rethinking stress: The role of mindsets in determining the stress response," *Journal of Personality and Social Psychology* 104 (2013): 716–33.

14. J. Blascovich, "Challenge and threat appraisal," in A. Elliot, ed., *Handbook of Approach and Avoidance Motivation* (New York, NY: Psychology Press, 2008), 431–45.

15. M. Babyak et al., "Exercise treatment for major depression: Maintenance of therapeutic benefit at 10 months," *Psychosomatic Medicine* 62 (2000): 633–38.

16. K. A. Ericcson and N. Charness, "Expert performance: Its structure and acquisition," *American Psychologist* 49 (1994): 725–47.

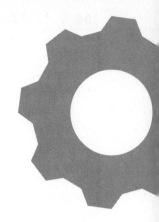

16 CAREER, LEARNING, AND SERVICE

BY W. JARED DUPREE, PHD, MBA

"WORK, LOVE AND PLAY ARE THE GREAT BALANCE WHEELS OF MAN'S BEING."[1] —ORISON SWETT MARDEN

In chapter 1, we discussed twelve different spokes in the Wheel of Wellness that influence our overall well-being. One of those layers includes the networks of people in our lives that make up our sense of community. These networks could include our friends or family, professional providers, school or work, church, neighbors, and more. We know that the people we include in our life and *how* we include them impacts our health and wellness. We also know that our choices of profession (or our main life roles) have a profound impact on overall health and happiness.

In this chapter, we will address why it is important to choose the right type of people in your support networks and how using the important people in your life can help build a more firm foundation of support. We will also discuss how the ways in which you engage in your career, in your education, and in giving back to others can either hurt or help your wellness.

Each of us is connected to the outside world in many ways. Many of us are employed or work from home, while some of us are involved in furthering our education. Many of us volunteer our time to participate in religious or charitable activities. These areas of our lives can provide us with resources, pleasure, and purpose. Or they can bring stress, displeasure, and dread. This chapter will provide you with some initial ideas for how to get the most out of your career, beginning with some observations about gaining an education and including some ideas for ways to integrate service as a method for finding happiness in your occupation and throughout your life.

The areas of my career that have brought the most anxiety to me have to do with money, time, balance and personal enjoyment. At times, I have wanted to make more money, have more time, not work so much, play more, and enjoy my work more. If that list sounds about as realistic as winning the lottery, you aren't alone. But with planning and intentional decision-making, you *can* make more money, work less, play more, and enjoy what you do—all at the same time.

BEGIN HERE: DEVELOP A CAREER PLAN

When the students I teach are beginning to consider their careers, I have them develop career plans that include one-, five-, ten-, twenty-, and forty-year plans, along with exit plans. I suggest the career plan include the following areas:

- **Family Considerations**. What type of hours do I want to work as I consider my family obligations? Do I want to live close to extended family? How much commute time is too much?

- **Finances**. How much will I need to earn to provide for my family's needs and wants?

- **Life Balance**. How many hours can I afford to devote to work and still have time left for other important pursuits? Am I okay with the idea of working long hours in a startup or entrepreneurial venture, or would I prefer a nine-to-five job?

- **Motivation**. Do I hunt until I find my passion, or can I bring passion to almost any kind of work? Is there an amount of time spent (or money earned) that is too much because it takes away from other areas of my life?

- **Talents and Skills**. How do my talents and skills align with my current position or future desired positions?

- **Education**. What season or stage of life am I in? Do I need more education or skills? How will I gain those skills?

- **Health and Wellness**. How will my work and finances impact my ability to exercise and live well? How much of my day will I be sedentary as opposed to active?

- **Work Environment**. What size of organization is important to me? What core values does this organization have, and how do they align with mine?

Discuss this plan with your significant other or with a life coach as needed. Some of you may be close to retirement or taking time away from work or even deciding not to work in a paid position. A career plan can include ways to volunteer, participate in charities and community events or organizations, and use your skills and talents in a meaningful way. As you develop your career plan, keep in mind three important considerations:

1. Remember your "why."

2. Remember your season.

3. Remember your place.

THE "WHY" BEHIND A CAREER

I remember one frustrating experience working with professionals in rural Mississippi who were discussing ways to help struggling clients change some of their destructive patterns. These professionals wanted us to discuss communications methods with these families in order to help them learn to manage their levels of stress. In reality, half of the families we were discussing had no idea where they were going to get food that night for their kids. A discussion of "I feel" statements certainly wasn't the thing these people needed. What they needed *most* to help manage stress levels was adequate food, a way to pay the rent, and some basic health care. What they needed *most* seemed to be good jobs. If our job is not helping us meet our basic needs, nothing else really matters. We need food today; we need to survive today. Thus, being employed in a career that provides for our financial needs can be critical to overall wellness.

Once basic needs are met, some of us are able to find life purpose, intrinsic motivation, psychological flow, or a deep sense of enjoyment in our career or job. This is not *necessary* to enjoy our jobs or do them well; however, we do know that people that enjoy their work for whatever reason tend to perform better. Researchers have discovered that the mind-set we have about our job is almost more important than what we are actually doing. For example, "Does the professional baseball player love to play baseball just as much as he did when he wasn't being paid?" Or, on an even deeper level, "Does the professional baseball player love baseball more than the guy that watches baseball on TV and plays locally for fun?" These are important questions. Recently, a friend of mine gave up professional golf as a career at the age of forty-two. He is making a permanent career change and says he thinks he may enjoy golf more now as a result.

Most of us can survive in an unpleasant job or can survive overwork for a short time, particularly if that job is preparing us to achieve higher goals, but what happens if you are feeling stuck or worry that you have chosen the wrong career? It may be helpful to realize that your career can fit your life purpose in different ways. Some will choose a career that will be based on performing a service or being involved in an industry they love. Others find their purpose in providing a product they are passionate about. Still others may discover that they really enjoy learning, and they gravitate to careers that allow for constant personal growth in a particular area or expertise.

On the other hand, you may not love your job much at all and will pursue your passions outside of your work, and your favorite learning and experiences will happen beyond the walls of your workplace. Can you still find satisfaction in your job? Absolutely.

For one, your job becomes a means to an end. Your career helps you earn the money needed to take care of your family, which will provide you with a sense of achievement. You may get a chance to work with people you enjoy being around. It may be that you choose your career because a unique work schedule allows you to engage in outside hobbies and interests. Maybe your employer offers flexible hours, work-from-home options, or project-based payment that gives autonomy you appreciate. Perhaps your job simply provides you with benefits that add some security to your life. Your motivation to be in your job and to do it well comes from a place within. Finding that motivation (the *why* behind your career choice) allows you to use your job as a tool to create heightened pleasure and joy in other areas of your life. For some of us, reframing or shifting our views of what a career or job means can do a lot to improve our outlook for how we engage in our work duties each day. When we find more meaning behind what we do, we are able to complete our duties and engage with others more effectively.

REMEMBER YOUR SEASON

About five years ago, I quit a great job to move closer to family. I was working in Houston, Texas, and really enjoyed my work. However, I realized at the time that if I didn't make a move now, that I would be living two thousand miles away from extended family for the next ten to fifteen years, and by that time, my kids may have missed important opportunities to get to know their grandparents, aunts, uncles, and cousins. I left Texas with a wife and three kids and no job prospects. It was a huge risk, but it was a season when I could afford to take a risk. Prior planning had left us with some savings we could live off from while I searched for new employment. I found purpose in the hope that my children would benefit in the long run. I was fortunate to find employment rather quickly and have developed a nice little niche in my part of the world doing what I love. I have more time, I make more money, *and* I am closer to family. I was able to make this kind of move because I did it during the right season.

I have not always been so fortunate. I remember living in Mexico with ten dollars in my pocket and no means to get money. I remember living with a six-month-old baby and young wife in Hattiesburg, Mississippi, working our tails off for minimum wage. I remember times in the past hating my job and feeling physical distress every time I had to go to work. We all have experienced the hardships of work. But it is important to remember that work has seasons. The young teen wants to earn some extra cash for the weekends, the twenty-four-year-old college student is paying her rent to get through school, the fifty-year-old is weighing the options between changing jobs to move closer to grandchildren or staying at a firm with a higher paycheck, and the seventy-five-year-old is grateful to get a job at the local hardware store because he is bored to death sitting at home. For each of us there is a season. The important lesson is to identify the season we are in and align our job or career to fit that season.

One of the most important phrases I tell myself often is, "My four-year-old boy will only be four years old once." Once he is five or fifteen, my season to enjoy him as a four-year-old will never return. For me, it is important to remember what is important during my particular season. Currently, I am thirty-eight years old with a wife and four kids. My oldest is fifteen years old and my youngest is two years old. My goal every day is to get home to be at dinner with my kids, have the weekends free to play, and go on frequent vacations with my family. My season is to be with my wife and kids as much as possible in these important years of their lives. Even today, I'm watching the clock as I write this chapter. I have so much to do, but tomorrow will come, and there will be another day. I could earn more money if I spent more time working, but I would lose the time I have with my family. Knowing this has helped give me a sense of urgency to place boundaries on my work schedule so I can avoid my built-in tendency to overwork. Realizing that I am in a season that will not last forever helps me to live in the moment and just keep moving forward.

Ask yourself, "What season are you in?" How does your current season fit the career or job that you have or want to have? What is important for you? Do you need to make a certain amount of money? Do you need to have a certain amount of time away from work? What is important to you during this season of your life? Remember, your career is one piece of the pie. These areas of your life are all connected. How you engage in your career can influence your health, relationships, and life enjoyment in a deep way.

REMEMBER YOUR PLACE (IDENTIFYING DIFFERENT ROLES YOU CAN PLAY IN THE WORKPLACE)

If you know why you have a job and you know the reason for your current season, then you will have a better understanding of your role or place. In other words, you will be able to make better decisions about your career, whether that means changing jobs, tweaking a current job, or solidifying a job.

Creativity and Flow

People are able to find a sense of place and fill a unique role in even the most mundane jobs. For example, a janitor may not find particular enjoyment in cleaning floors and restrooms, but she may discover that she is especially talented at interacting with the children she sees at school. One university custodian found his "place" when he discovered that he could intersperse tedious jobs with more creative tasks no one else could do, like repairing cabinetry or designing and building an organizing rack for sports equipment. He was able to attend lectures during his breaks, and he enjoyed the opportunity to have brief, but meaningful religious and political discussions with his colleagues who were professors. Access to those "fringe benefits" made the job much less mundane. Someone working out of doors may find pleasure in being in nature, while someone in an office setting may find enjoyment in forming connections with coworkers. Similar to finding your life purpose, part of your success in your career is found through an alignment with finding your place—discovering opportunities to employ your creativity and experience "flow" by creating new ideas, products, services, or relationships.

The key message here is to find your place by aligning your talents and interests with the areas in your job that are most in harmony with those talents and interests. Flow and creativity will follow, leading to more enjoyment and success.

Trust

My dissertation focused on figuring out what factors help people to be extremely successful in their careers. I examined transcripts from interviews and conducted my own interviews with scientists, actors, musicians, businesspeople, clinicians, and pioneers, and I discovered that improved innovation and success is fostered when coworkers are able to develop trust. Leaders who exhibited integrity, interpersonal skills, appropriate self-disclosure, proactivity, common vision and motivations, and sincerity had more success and enjoyment in their workplace, both because they were trustworthy and because they were able to build trust among others. An effective organization recognizes an employee with the ability to build trust and treats that person like gold because this individual will help the company innovate and succeed.

As you consider your place or role, consider how you can improve your ability to build trust with others. For example, Doug, a sales manager, might build trust with his sales representatives by getting to know them, serving them, mentoring their efforts to build their list of clients and increase commissioned earnings, being honest with them, and complimenting their efforts. This level of trust will likely be a key to success for the sales team because each representative can trust his or her manager to do what is best. You may not always like your actual duties, but you always have a chance to work with others and build trust. As you do, your value rises along with your effectiveness and enjoyment. In fact, many organizations and corporations have listed the ability to build trust with others as their number one need for future employees.

Work-Life Connection

We know that what we do in the workplace transfers over to what we do in our personal lives. We know how much we enjoy our work and what we do for a living impacts our physical health, mental health, mood, energy levels, relationships, stress management, and life balance. We know that if work isn't going well, discontentment is likely to bleed into other areas of our lives. Remembering our place in work is also about remembering our place in life.

Your role at work may be to spend extra hours getting your new startup off the ground, or it may be decreasing your work hours so that you can get home and cook healthier meals for yourself. Your role at work may be to simplify your work so you can focus effort and energy building your role in a different area of your life. There may not be a need to aggressively progress or "move up the ladder" in the office because it is more important to "move up the ladder" in your role as a mother or father.

Equally, learning how to handle stress or deal with difficult relationships at work can prepare us to handle stress at home or work through challenges with a difficult teenager or challenging neighbor. Thus, remembering our place reminds us that work is only one piece of the big picture.

Being mindful about your work may mean you need to step back and gain some perspective by asking yourself what is most important right now in your life—the bigger paycheck or more time with an aging parent. It is possible that you will discover that you need to perform well at work only to a point so that you'll have time and energy left to perform spectacularly well in another area of your life.

In summary, remembering the *why* behind your career (discovering for yourself why it is that you work), remembering your *season* (discovering the best time and place for your work) and remembering your *place* in your work (bringing passion to your work through nurturing creativity, building trust, and setting priorities) are three keys to a career that will bring you significant pleasure.

Retirement

I do want to mention a few ideas about retirement. In many ways, retirement is just another stage of your career—except you generally don't get paid during this stage of your career. In other words, if you have a mind-set that work is an area that allows you to connect with others, learn, grow, create, progress, and provide for other roles in your life, then retirement will likely offer the same advantages. You will need to consider how to replace certain duties or titles, but in general, you will likely discover that happy retirement is similar to happy work. Align your interests and passions with your activities. Find purpose in what you do. Connect with others. Remember the big picture.

Education and Learning

I have discovered that education and learning aren't always the same thing. We do know that helping people learn a new skill or hobby adds to life enjoyment; we also know that learning a new hobby together with a spouse or friend adds even more enjoyment. Educating yourself with the purpose of obtaining a degree or certification so you can find a job is only part of educating yourself. Here are a few thoughts to consider as you decide how to balance your life with learning and education:

Consider getting a college degree for a job versus a college degree merely for learning and exploration.

Unfortunately, many students earn a degree and then try to fit a job to that degree. Instead, I encourage students to find a job or set of jobs they enjoy and earn a degree that provides them with the skills and tools for those jobs.

I have found that students are much more motivated and enjoy the learning process more when they freely explore who they are first and *then* commit to a particular degree or course of study based on what they learn about themselves.

Learning comes in many forms.

The education you receive through colleges, universities, and technical schools is only one of many forms of learning. I have relatives and friends who have earned the highest degree possible in their fields of study yet are currently doing something entirely unrelated as a career. I have relatives who have never earned a college degree yet are extremely successful in entrepreneurial endeavors. I know others that are avid readers and know more about their "hobby" subject than someone that has a degree in the same area of study. I know people who have earned a degree from a particular school that opened doors to opportunities they wouldn't have gained otherwise. There are many paths to learning and obtaining a job. There are even more paths to learning for the sake of learning itself.

When I was eighteen, I was interested in reading biographies and autobiographies for a time. I remember reading the autobiographies of Isaac Asimov and Louis L'amour. They both listed the number of books they had read from their early days to the present, mainly focusing on key titles that influenced them. They were avid readers, and they read all types of books. Neither of them read only books from the genre they eventually wrote in. More of us should follow their example.

When I was in Edinburgh, Scotland, I decided to take a couple of community classes in the evening on swing dancing. My wife and I have competed in swing dancing in the past, and I had learned that swing dancing in Scotland was an active and vibrant pastime for all ages. My wife wanted me to learn some new moves to bring home and teach her, so I went hesitantly to a location in Edinburgh, thinking I may be too old. I was pleasantly surprised to see people of all ages from eighteen to seventy-five using the traditional teaching format of switching partners every couple of minutes or so. I had a great time and brought home some new moves! I have personally found that learning something like swing dancing with my wife has added a lot to my life enjoyment. Equally, I enjoy learning areas of interests with my kids together. My daughter loves to cook, and we pull out recipes to try. My son loves to mountain bike, and we go out often. Even my infant daughter loves animals, and I try to find opportunities to indulge her interest in bears and kitties. Learning can be a connecting process as we grow in a new area together. Consider learning a new hobby or sharing a hobby with someone else.

Finally, I am a big proponent of learning through meeting different peoples and cultures. I travel often and enjoy meeting the locals. I have played soccer ("futbol") on the beaches of La Llorona, Mexico, with the native people. I have worked side by side in the Andes, building concrete block homes. I have sweated in the sauna with European friends. I have seen the poverty of the Appalachians, I have seen the wealth of large country estates, and I have eaten some of the best seafood I've ever tasted out of a gas station in the backwoods of Louisiana. I really enjoy getting to know the depth of people and the way they live beyond the touristy locations. I have discovered the more I learn about others, the more I learn about myself. We are all connected in the end. We all live on this one planet and are brothers and sisters.

Learn for life.

A friend of mine who researches the impact of relationships on dementia mentioned to me the importance of learning and learning together as a measure for preventing or slowing the progress of dementia. In addition, learning through physical exercise and hobbies has also been shown to help prevent or slow down the process of muscle and joint issues like arthritis and osteoporosis. In general, keeping our minds and bodies active, alert, and learning will help prevent and slow down disease as well as provide life enjoyment benefits. Making sure we stay connected to nature or feeding our soul through music, art, and spirituality will add to the creativity, purpose, and love we have for life and others.

Give service.

We know that volunteering and giving service leads to reports of higher life satisfaction, lower mortality rates, better mental health and better physical health.[2] The research suggests that even though volunteering is beneficial to all ages, older adults show greater benefits in both their health and sense of well-being. Erik Erikson, a psychologist, developed a theory addressing life stages that each of us experiences. He suggests that each life stage provides us with challenges that are meant to be overcome. As we overcome these challenges, we learn valuable tools and skills that will aid us in the next stage. Thus, one stage builds on the other as we develop and grow. The last stage in his theory is called *Integrity versus Despair*. In this stage, older adults reflect on their lives and consider their victories and defeats. Integrity is gained through the wisdom of accepting the good, the bad, and the ugly of life. This wisdom leads to a giving back attitude. Although volunteerism and service have been researched more among older adults, we do know that people that offer service in general report higher levels of life satisfaction.

We also know that giving service is a way to practice mindfulness—especially when giving is in the form of physical labor. There is a sense of peace and serenity of engaging in a physical activity that is not connected to any stress of finances, job, or duty. The freedom to engage in the labor with no return or responsibility provides the mind with serenity.

When someone freely gives services out of love for others or a higher power, the service itself is freeing. The importance of autonomy and freedom, along with motivation, seems to be important as we give service. We must choose to serve out of a desire to help or grow if we are to make the most of this area in our lives, and we must balance the level of service we perform if we are to keep our own lives in balance.

I have worked with individuals who give so much time to their church that their family is struggling at home. Others discover that adding service to a busy routine actually helps inform their choice of priorities, making it easier to let go of other busy tasks that were crowding out things that were more important. For example, a mother who is forced to give up a volunteer opportunity in order to stay home with a critically ill child may find that she doesn't miss being PTA president at all but relishes playing in the backyard with her children in the evenings instead.

It is important to know when to say yes and when to say no to be able to fully serve. Choose areas of community service that touch your heart and align with your passions and talents.

ACTION ITEMS

1. **Develop a career plan**. Develop a career plan that includes one-, five-, ten-, twenty-, and forty-year plans, along with exit plans. If you are in a dead-end job or you are pursuing a degree without considering what career you'll pursue once the diploma is in hand, take time to visit with a career counselor and start looking at options available to you. Discover your own why, your own season, and your favorite role as you consider a career move.

2. **Learn a new hobby or share a hobby with someone.** Consider learning a new hobby or talent by yourself or with someone. If you are married, consider learning a new hobby with your spouse.

3. **Always be reading a good book or two.** This is a simple one. Always have a book or two that you can read weekly, if not daily. I always keep a great book on my nightstand. Choose contemporary and classic pieces as well as areas that you enjoy to get a well-rounded education.

4. **Choose to serve in your own way.** Remember, it is important to freely choose to serve, without compulsion from outside forces. Decide how you are going to serve each week, whether that is part of a formal group or through an informal desire to help a family member

or friend. Consider adding ways to serve each week, especially as you consider ways to help you learn, grow, and connect.

CONCLUSION

As you consider ways to connect with your community and the roles you have outside of your home, it is important to align who you are with what you do. As you consider your career or ways that you volunteer and serve, it is important to remember how to take advantage of your time in this life. Each stage of life provides us with challenges and opportunities. Sometimes we can let our job or work take precedence over other areas of our life. Sometimes our work can deeply impact us which can bleed over to other parts of our lives. Because we can only control what we can control, I have found that attempting to increase autonomy, learning, creativity, and personal alignment with respect to career, community, and areas of service leads to more success and enjoyment. This doesn't mean that challenges, failures, and boredom go away; it means we have a better sense of what to do with them when they come.

NOTES

1.   Orison Swett Marden, as quoted in Brett Dupree *Joyous Expansion: Unleashing Your Passions to Achieve an Inspired Life* (Portland, OR: BookBaby, 2014).

2.   R. Grimm, K. Spring, and N. Dietz, "The health benefits of volunteering: A review of recent research," The Office of Research & Policy Development: Washington, DC, 2007.

17 FINANCES AND WELLNESS

RACQUEL HEATH TIBBETS, MBA, CFP®, CPA;
KRISTY ARCHULETA, PHD, LMFT; & HANNAH RICE

"KNOW WHAT YOU OWN AND WHY YOU OWN IT."[1] —PETER LYNCH

RACQUEL HEATH TIBBETTS, MBA, CFP®, CPA, is the *vice president and senior financial planner with Key Private Bank in New England. Racquel has been providing Key clients with comprehensive and customized financial solutions since 1999. Prior to joining Key, Racquel was an accountant for Berry, Dunn, McNeil & Parker, a CPA firm headquartered in Maine. She earned her bachelor's degree in business administration and MBA from the University of Maine in Orono. She also earned her CPA certificate from the State of Maine in 2003 and CFP® certificate in 2008. Racquel is a PhD student at Kansas State University in the personal financial planning program. Racquel currently resides in North Yarmouth, Maine.*

KRISTY ARCHULETA, PhD. *Her career objective is to bridge financial planning and family therapy to form a type of financial therapy, where financial planners and relationship therapists work together to provide comprehensive treatment to clients experiencing financial distress. Her research interests include rural and farm families, dyadic processes influencing financial satisfaction and marital satisfaction, empirical-based treatment for couples experiencing financial difficulties, and theoretical development to understand the connections between financial planning and couple relationships and how to work with them. Dr. Archuleta is a licensed marriage and family therapist in the state of Kansas and an associate professor at Kansas State University.*

HANNAH RICE, BA, *is a student in the personal financial planning program at Kansas State University. She is an active member in Kansas States' chapter of the Financial Planning Association. She has a passion for learning—particularly where money meets different areas of our lives.*

217

KYRA'S STORY

I have been making my own choices on how I spend my money and time for nearly twenty years. These choices were significantly influenced by my parents, teachers, friends, society, and media. It is easy to reflect on that now and even place blame when things didn't go well financially. I took out the maximum student loan debt I could while in my first five years of college, which was about five times what I actually needed to pay for tuition and books. And since I had a job that paid pretty well, I had an expensive lifestyle for that period of time. When I finally made it to graduation, I was lucky I had a job, because it was time to pay back those loans. In fact, I am still paying on those loans.

I spent the early years after graduation working and spending almost everything I was making. I was fortunate that my education and degree was in accounting and business, so I knew the importance of contributing to the company retirement plan and did so at least up to the match. I didn't think much about my health. I had health insurance. I didn't think much about what I was consuming or how much.

That all changed one day when I hurt my knee. I went to the doctor's office and told the receptionist why I was there. She ordered an X-ray, and while I was sitting in the office waiting for an X-ray technician, I became concerned about whether or not my insurance was going to cover the cost. I called my insurance company and was told that my estimated out-of-pocket cost for an X-ray was about $300. Well, I didn't have an extra $300, so I asked the receptionist if I really needed an X-ray. She told me that I had the option to see the doctor first. Gosh, that made too much sense! When I saw the doctor, he told me an X-ray was unnecessary and that my knee injury and future knee injuries could be prevented if I would lose twenty pounds. Ouch!

With that experience, things started to make more sense to me: I have twenty-four hours in a day. I was earning $35,000 a year. This is what I had to work with. I needed a budget for my money and my time. I didn't want to have to spend any of it on medical bills and therefore needed to do whatever I could to get healthy and stay healthy. Consequently, part of my money was spent on a gym membership and healthier food choices. Part of my time was and still is spent on exercise, and part of my time was spent learning and understanding what I should be eating and drinking. It's a bit of an oversimplification, but if you can add and subtract, you can do it.

This time and money plan has been part of me ever since, through houses, a marriage, job changes, and kids. One of the biggest rewards has been good mental health, evidenced by lower stress and an improved ability to overcome life's challenges. There are so many ways that stress from health issues and money problems can affect us. This testimonial is an example of how health, finances, and overall wellness are integrated.

WHAT IS FINANCIAL WELLNESS?

Money is the number one stressor for Americans.[2] This finding should come as no surprise because money is everywhere in our daily lives. It is used for basic survival: to eat, stay warm, and keep a roof over our heads. We use it to have fun: to go to a movie, out to dinner, or to an amusement park. Money factors into nearly every aspect of our lives, either directly or indirectly. Whether a person is rich or poor, finances impact our psychological, relational, and physical health.

Financial wellness, also known as financial well-being (we'll use the terms interchangeably in this chapter), includes both objective and subjective factors, including financial status, financial satisfaction, financial stress, financial attitudes, financial knowledge, and financial behaviors.[3, 4] Subjectively, we measure financial wellness in terms of positive and negative psychological reactions to our own financial situation: "I was elated when my boss gave me a raise" or, "My wife's refusal to stick to a budget infuriates me." Objectively, financial wellness can be measured numerically by evaluating cash flow (income versus expenses) and net worth (assets versus debt).

Why is financial wellness important? Financial wellness has been found to be a solid predictor of overall wellness. It stands to reason that economic distress has been found to be an important determinant of psychological well-being.[5] Yet the old adage that money doesn't buy happiness is actually true. Research tells us that the level of income isn't what contributes to life satisfaction. Rather, life satisfaction depends on whether a family's financial needs are met. When a family's financial obligations are met, then happiness peaks. You may be surprised to learn that the income a family receives *beyond* meeting financial needs does not necessarily improve happiness. In other words, once your basic needs are met, more money does *not* mean you'll be happier.

So why do we stress so much about making more money and getting ahead? Here are some thoughts:

1. **Higher income is associated with more successful life outcomes**. A higher education is typically associated with a greater amount of income. Higher income and higher education level can lead to better family outcomes. When parents have higher income and a higher level of education, their children are likely to have fewer behavior and academic problems.[6]

2. **Higher income has been found to be related to better health** but also that better health led to higher wealth,[7] meaning that money and health can be seen as cyclical. This makes sense, especially when considering Bloom and Canning's explanation about how healthier populations have higher labor productivity because they can work more, which can result in higher income. These populations develop their skills through education. When people have better health, they live longer, allowing them the time to further develop skills. The income of the population increases because there are more people in the workforce. This continues the cycle from better health to higher productivity to higher income.

3. **Poor health hinders the ability to work**, and it can also lead to medical bills. Unpaid medical bills can lead to reductions in savings, increases in other debt, and even bankruptcy.[8, 9] Unpaid medical bills are a leading cause of bankruptcies,[10] regardless of whether a person has insurance. According to a study by the Center for Studying Health System Change (HSC), about twenty million American families (approximately forty-three million people) reported problems paying medical bills in 2003, despite the fact that two-thirds of these families reported having medical insurance.[11]

PRINCIPLES OF FINANCIAL WELLNESS

What we now know about money is that it is interrelated with a whole host of other wellness factors. So much so that money, or the lack of it, can sometimes be a significant driving factor for improving or destroying an individual's overall sense of wellness. Consider Kyra's story at the outset of this chapter. Her problem was not just a physical problem with her knee; it was also a problem that affected her financial and psychological wellness. What if Kyra was married or in a serious relationship? Would her injured knee, her worries about paying for X-rays, and the lifestyle changes she implemented in order to address the doctor's proposed weight loss have had an impact with her partner? They could have.

Relational Health

You probably know a couple who fights about money. If you think that you do not know a couple who fights about money, then they just have not told you they fight about money. Money is the common issue that couples fight about, along with parenting and sex.[12] In fact, money is one of the most intensely fought about issues in relationships and financial conflict is a strong predictor of divorce.[13, 14]

Why is money so stressful to individuals and relationships? Because it is an emotionally charged issue. We all have attitudes and beliefs about money that we absorb from the communities around us. These attitudes and beliefs are developed in childhood and based on direct and indirect messages about money that were sent by parents, extended family members, friends, school, and media.[15] Consider how emotionally-charged some of the following statements might be, depending on your point of view:

- "You can't take it with you, so I would just as soon buy the $250 designer jeans."

- "Overdrafting the bank account isn't a problem as long as you have overdraft protection."

- "I'm saving up for a rainy day, so I decided not to get you an anniversary gift this year."

- "He thinks we should buy a four-wheeler, but everyone knows a piano is a better investment."

Money is often seen as a taboo topic to discuss in a family and especially with people outside of the family, making feelings about money difficult to process. The lack of being aware about our feelings toward money can result in emotionally reacting to money issues when they arise in our interpersonal relationships. This emotionally charged reaction can override our rational way of thinking and interacting in an intimate relationship when the topic of money arises and when financial goals and values differ. The outcome is a conflict that can quickly escalate in a way that positive communication and resolution skills are tossed out, intensifying the strain between partners. If Kyra had been married and had chosen to continue with her unhealthy lifestyle, resulting in medical bills and psychological stress, then she and her husband may have found their marital relationship in distress.

Psychological Health

We saw how Kyra's story at the beginning of this chapter could be related to psychological health. She made choices that improved her financial wellness, and those decisions continue to impact her overall wellness. But it's also easy to see how a different set of choices may have produced a different psychological outcome. Indeed, research shows that negative financial factors can lower self-confidence, provoke depression symptoms, and even increase thoughts of suicide. Emotional pain like depression and anxiety can be triggered by financial factors like lower socioeconomic status, economic distress, income, debt, and bankruptcy.[16]

Consider the following scenario, for example: Harry's business went bankrupt, and his wife became so distressed that she lost her appetite. She was so embarrassed by the bankruptcy, she stopped going to social events and lay sleepless in her bed for weeks at a time, worrying about how they would ever fund their retirement.

Physical Health

When finances become shaky enough, a downward spiral of health and financial woes is almost inevitable. For example, a single parent of three children is already emotionally stressed and worried if she struggles to make sure her family has enough to eat. Her situation continues to decline as she loses her job and has no family that can afford to take her and her kids in. This stress then leads to an ulcer in her stomach. She develops type 2 diabetes due to coping with the stress she has experienced for years by emotionally overeating junk food. These physical problems lead back to financial problems due to her inability to pay medical bills, further raising anxiety.

This example explains how the aspects of financial, psychological, and financial distress are cyclical. Furthermore, if this mom has a partner, any of these stressors could negatively affect the couple relationship, adding to the cyclical nature of her physical and financial problems.

WHAT CAN WE DO TO BE FINANCIALLY WELL?

What should you do to reach financial wellness? Begin by thinking about what you want your financial future to look like. Next, identify short-term (less than one year), medium-term (one to five years) and long-term goals (beyond five years) that will help you achieve your financial goal. Then write these goals down and make them specific. This is a good time to implement the SMART goal strategy.[17]

Specific: I'll reduce my credit card debt.

Measurable: I'll reduce from $3,000 to $0.

Achievable: I know I can reach this goal by cutting up my credit card so I don't add to the debt, and then earn extra income by doing ten hours of overtime work per month and selling my stereo system.

Realistic: I'll create an expectation for myself I know I can actually achieve.

Time-bound: I'll have my credit card balance completely paid twelve months from now.

For example, a SMART goal would breakdown the typical goal of eliminating card debt to state, "I will reduce by $3,000 credit card debt to $0 within the next twelve months." You want your goal to be so clearly stated that it's easy to confirm whether you accomplished it or not.

To help develop your goals as a way to reach your ideal financial future, you may need to enlist some of the following strategies.

Evaluate Objective Financial Wellness

To gain an overall picture of your financial situation, it is important to evaluate your money. The hard numbers do not lie.

1. Track your fixed and variable expenses for four weeks. Fixed expenses are the bills you have every month that do not change like rent or a mortgage, car payment, and utilities. Variable expenses fluctuate from month to month and can range from buying groceries to buying a soda from the vending machine.

2. After you have tracked how much you spend each month, you can develop a spending plan that will help you estimate how much you plan to spend each month. By keeping simple records, you'll be able to compare to how you actually spent your money once the month is over by checking your bank statements and other records.

3. If you estimate that you spend more than your income, then look for ways that you can reduce expenses. What are you willing to do different to not exceed your income? If you see a shortfall coming, how will you handle it? Do you have an emergency fund? Experts recommend that an emergency fund should hold savings equal to three to six months of expenses, in the case that you or your partner (if a couple) loses their job. The emergency fund can also be used for unexpected expenses like when a car breaks down and it has to be fixed or the refrigerator dies. If three to six months of expenses seems unrealistic right now, start by working toward saving a smaller amount, like $500. Once you reach that goal, work toward saving $1000, and then toward $1500, and so on.

4. Developing a net worth statement is another important financial tool. Net worth statements identify assets (what you own) and debts

(what you owe). Net worth is considered to be a snapshot of a person's financial situation. Net worth typically increases over a person's lifetime. Generally, younger people have lower net worth because they have more financial obligations like mortgages and student loans and have not had a chance to build their assets like savings in a retirement account or outright ownership of a home. Tools like financial ratios can be used with budgets and net worth statements to measure an individual's financial health when compared to a standard benchmark.

Develop Communication and Conflict Resolution Skills

Trust is the foundation to any relationship and is also central to financial wellness in a couple relationship. Eighty percent of individuals keep secrets about money from their partners. Secrets may range from buying a new pair of shoes to having a bank account that the partner does not know about. These types of secrets could damage a couple's relationship. Maintaining trust can be facilitated through open and honest communication and solid conflict resolutions skills. If you cannot talk about money with each other and you do not know how to resolve conflict, money will be a constant source of stress in your relationship.

Although it is helpful for couples to be on the same page in terms of financial goals and values,[18] *how* a couple communicates about money is really the key. John Gottman's research on couple relationships has helped to demystify harmful communication. Gottman can predict with almost perfect precision (91 percent accuracy) whether a couple will end up divorcing in the future based on how they talk to each other.[19] He suggests that couples who engage in criticism, contempt (name-calling, eye-rolling, and so on), defensiveness (blaming), and stonewalling (avoiding or ignoring) are at higher risk of divorce. Because money is an emotionally charged issue and financial satisfaction and relationship satisfaction are closely tied,[20] learning positive communication and money management skills may be critical to maintaining a healthy marriage. If you and your partner have experienced a significant amount of conflict over finances and have not been successful finding healthy ways to talk about money, don't delay reaching out for help.

Utilize Professional Resources

Traditionally, money has been thought of as a topic that is solely numeric and to be left to financial planners and counselors. However, research over the past decade has demonstrated that money expands beyond the expertise of financial professionals. Mental health clinicians have long seen individuals and families present money-related issues to therapy. With little training in finances, mental health professionals often ignore the money-related problems and hope that the money problems get better if other problem areas are improved. On the flip side, financial professionals have begun to recognize that their clients' interpersonal and intrapersonal relationships affect financial behaviors and financial decision making, which have an impact on overall quality of life.[21] Recognizing the need for therapists to combine both skill sets (financial wisdom plus the ability to provide emotional counseling) to improve financial well-being, experts have begun to develop an emerging field known as financial therapy.

Because it is such a new field, there is no certification system yet to identify professionals who practice financial therapy. However, financial planners, counselors, coaches, and mental health therapists may each practice aspects of financial therapy. This field will continue to evolve and progress, but in the meantime, working with a professional may be the next step you need to take in order to improve or even maintain your financial health.

Sometimes, professional help is thought of as something to fix your problems. However, it is just as important to maintain financial wellness. Finding the right professionals in your community can be tricky, but it is important to identify what it is that you need and what you want to accomplish and then find those people who can help you. Here is a list of some of the professional certifications to consider when searching for help:

- *Certified financial planners*™ can help you develop your goals, create a spending plan, help you get organized, and encourage you stay on track. They typically integrate tax, insurance, investments, retirement, and estate planning to develop a comprehensive financial plan that focuses on reaching long-term financial goals.

- *Accredited financial counselors*® can help in resolving financial problems like credit card debt and student loans. They can help you set financial goals and develop a spending plan to meet typically short- to mid-term goals.

- *Mental health clinicians* such as licensed marriage and family therapists, clinical psychologists, clinical social workers, and professional counselors who work with money-related issues can help with subjective factors in order to help change behavior as a way to reach financial wellness. These professionals are typically regulated by state law and can diagnose and treat dysfunctional behavior. Often, health insurance can be used to help pay for these services.

Although this is not an exhaustive list of credentialed professionals, any one of the professional groups listed may incorporate financial therapy into their practice. Financial therapy is an emerging field of practice and study that integrates cognitive, emotional, relational, and economic factors to improve financial well-being. The Financial Therapy Association (FTA) houses the FTA Network, which lists professionals who have identified themselves as financial therapists or professionals who do financial therapy–related work. You can learn more at FinancialTherapyAssociation.org.

When searching for a professional who may be of assistance to you, take time to interview them. Ask them how they define financial wellness, what approach they use to work toward improving or helping a person maintain financial wellness, and about their fee structure. Look for professionals who work with both the subjective and the objective factors related to financial wellness. Be leery of financial professionals who work only off of commission. Their goal is typically to sell you something. In addition, be wary of for-profit-debt management companies. These companies also use a commission system, and typically they only do for you what you can do for yourself.

CONCLUSION

Financial wellness is a gift that you can give yourself. It is not based solely on your income. It's more a function of taking control of your relationship with money. Start by envisioning your ideal financial future and what financial wellness looks like to you. Then assess your resources and examine your own money beliefs. Based on your resources, identify goals that you can meet and are able to identify when the goal has been completed. Try some of the strategies above to help reach your financial goals. Do not be afraid to change your behaviors in order to improve your financial wellness. Kyra did it; so can you!

NOTES

1. Peter Lynch, as quoted in "Peter Lynch's Principles & Golden Rules of Investing," September 18, 2012, http://www.marketfolly.com/2012/09/peter-lynchs-principles-golden-rules-of.html.

2. American Psychological Association, "The impact of stress [Press release]," 2006, http://www.apa.org/news/press/releases/stress/2012/impact.aspx?item=2.

3. S. Joo, "Personal financial wellness" in J. J. Xiao, ed., *Handbook of Consumer Finance Research* (New York, NY: Springer, 2008), 21–33.

4. Aimee D. Prawitz et al., "InCharge financial distress/financial well-being scale: Development, administration, and score interpretation," *Journal of Financial Counseling and Planning* 17, no. 1 (2006).

5. R. J. Mills et al., "The effects of gender, family satisfaction, and economic strain on psychological well-being," *Family Relations* (1992): 440–45.

6. Melissa A. Milkie, Kei M. Nomaguchi, and Kathleen E. Denny, "Does the Amount of Time Mothers Spend With Children or Adolescents Matter?" *Journal of Marriage and Family* 77, no. 2 (2015): 355–72.

7. D. Bloom and D. Canning, "The Health and Wealth of Nations" 287 (2000): 1–3.

8. B. O'Neill et al., "Financially distressed consumers: Their financial practices, financial well-being, and health," *Financial Counseling and Planning* 16 (2005): 73–88.

9. R. W. Seifert and M. Rukavina, "Bankruptcy is the tip of a medical-debt iceberg," *Health Affairs* 25, no. 2 (2006): w89–w92.

10. D. Himmelstein et al., "Medical Bankruptcy in the United States, 2007: Results of a National Study," *The American Journal of Medicine* 122, no. 8 (2007): 1–6.

11. J. H. May, and P. J. Cunningham, "Tough trade-offs: Medical bills, family finances and access to care," Center for Studying Health System Change, 2004, 85.

12. Lauren M. Papp, E. Mark Cummings, and Marcie C. Goeke-Morey, "For richer, for poorer: Money as a topic of marital conflict in the home," *Family Relations* 58, no. 1 (2009): 91–103.

13. Ibid.

14. Jeffrey Dew, Sonya Britt, and Sandra Huston, "Examining the relationship between financial issues and divorce," *Family Relations* 61, no. 4 (2012): 615–28.

15. Brad Klontz, Rick Kahler, and Ted Klontz, *Facilitating financial health: Tools for financial planners, coaches, and therapists* (Cincinnati, OH: National Underwriter Company, 2008).

16. Kristy L. Archuleta et al., "Financial satisfaction and financial stressors in marital satisfaction," *Psychological Reports* 108, no. 2 (2011): 563–76.

17. George T. Doran, "There's a S.M.A.R.T. Way to Write Management's Goals and Objectives," *Management Review*, 1981.

18. Kristy L. Archuleta, John E. Grable, and Sonya L. Britt, "Financial and relationship satisfaction as a function of harsh start-up and shared goals and values," *Journal of Financial Counseling and Planning* 24, no. 1 (2013): 4.

19. John Mordechai Gottman, *The Marriage Clinic: A Scientifically-Based Marital Therapy* (New York: WW Norton & Company, 1999).

20. Glen H. Elder et al., "Families under economic pressure," *Journal of Family Issues* 13, no. 1 (1992): 5–37.

21. Kristy L. Archuleta et al., "What is financial therapy? Discovering mechanisms and aspects of an emerging field," *Journal of Financial Therapy* 3, no. 2 (2012): 9.

SECTI⚙N
6

PLANNING FOR THE
REST OF YOUR LIFE

"The important thing to you is not how many years in your life, but how much life in your years!"

—Chicago Tribune *advertisement for* The Second Forty Years *by Edward J. Stieglitz, MD*

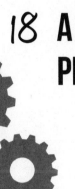
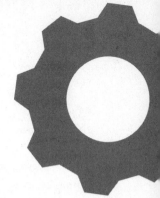

18 A PERSONAL LIFESTYLE PLAN FOR WELLNESS

BY W. JARED DUPREE, PHD, MBA

"SOMETIMES WE ARE MEANT TO COMFORT THE AFFLICTED;
SOMETIMES WE ARE MEANT TO AFFLICT THE COMFORTABLE."
—UNKNOWN

We have presented a lot of good information about different elements of wellness up to this point. As you can see, it is impossible to address all factors of wellness simultaneously. In fact, there are additional topics I could have added to this book, but to be concise, I've chosen to include the areas I think are most critical to an individual's overall wellness.

If you remember from chapter 2, we use a systemic lens at WholeFIT to consider how everything is connected. Each of the elements presented thus far fit together, influence one another, and ultimately can work in harmony to improve wellness and life enjoyment. At this point, you should be able to identify many of the wellness puzzle pieces that have a strong impact on your personal health and well-being. You may have a better sense of where you are strong and where you need additional support. How will you put all of the pieces together to craft a new master wellness plan for yourself?

Let's start with a quick review: In chapter 1 we presented the following diagrams to help us visually consider the different factors of wellness and how they influence one another. In Figure 1, we recognize how each of the following elements impact our wellness:

- body

- mind

- emotion

- spirit

- relationships

- leisure

- work

- community

In Figure 2, we recognize how these different elements may be influencing one another. For example, our relationships with our spouse, family, and a higher power influence our physical health. Our physical health influences our mood, thoughts, and motivation. Our life patterns impact our relationships. As discussed, each of these elements influence one another in a circular format. There is no one single cause. There is no silver bullet or magic pill. The key to living a well life is understanding how to take advantage of what we have (body, mind, spirit), know how to connect with others (partners, family, work, community) and have a life that allows us to grow in our various roles and ambitions (love, passions, hobbies, life purpose).

Because we are each different, the way we connect these principles and components is different for each person. The way we connect these elements will change over time. A young mother will have a different wellness plan than a retired husband. An ambitious executive will be different than a woman struggling with lupus. We are each different. We live in different stages. We each have different circumstances.

Your first impression for how to craft your own personal WholeFit wellness plan will probably be to place renewed emphasis on making positive changes in one of the areas in your life where you feel you may be struggling. It is likely an area that you have attempted to change over and over again. As you may already know, trying to open that same door of change the same way will likely get you the same result—it will remain closed. You need to try another door. In other words, the thing you are trying to fix may not be the thing that needs fixing at all.

As a clinician, I find that the people I am trying to help know exactly which areas they are struggling with the most. They will be the areas of wellness that you scored lower on when you filled out the integration wheel (see page 11). What most people fail to understand is that *solving* those weaknesses can sometimes be counterintuitive, and that's why you've never quite mastered a change, despite your almost desperate efforts to do so. A WholeFIT approach helps you see there may be a different door you can go through that leads to the change that you have been seeking.

Consider this example: I was working with a teen who was addicted to marijuana. He and his father were having a difficult time, while he and his mother had a pretty good relationship. The father had taken on the role of disciplinarian and struggled to communicate with his son. Instead of suggesting that they sit down and work on communication techniques, we tried a different approach. I had the father ask his son for advice about how to manage some of the father's stressors and frustrations at work. It started out slowly. The teen just would not engage that much. However, the father continued to ask about various situations rather than just asking if the son had done his homework or cleaned his room. Eventually, the teen began to share his opinion, and the father was surprised how spot-on his son's ideas were. He actually found much of the advice helpful. Soon, the teenager started asking the father for advice, which floored Dad. The greatest moment was when the father was able to ask, "I am struggling with knowing how to be a good father. I love my children and want what is best for them, but sometimes I get angry and say things I wish I didn't. I want to help them but don't want to feel like I did with my own father. He seemed only concerned about what other people thought. I want to have fun with them, but I get worried about their lives and sometimes miss opportunities. What should I do?" There is no way the father would have asked this question three months prior. He had too much fear and pride. Now, they had developed a relationship that allowed Dad to ask a question that pushed them past the "tipping point," and they developed a great relationship. Magically, the marijuana use went away.

It almost always surprises the client who comes to talk about his or her weight issues that I don't start with a focus on diet and exercise. The husband whose relationship with his wife has disintegrated is sometimes confused when I suggest we focus our efforts on his job satisfaction instead of focusing on the couple's problems in the bedroom. But this is the genius and the magic behind WholeFIT. Once we examine the whole person—the big picture, we can discover a new method of attack. We can approach the problem by going in a different door—one you've never tried before. And it can be incredibly hopeful to believe that there is a new way to succeed just waiting to be discovered.

Because I cannot sit down across the desk from most of my readers, I'll try to do the next best thing and show you examples of how I might help a person struggling in one of the following areas. With these examples in place, I'm hopeful you'll have some ideas for new approaches to try as you work to improve your own wellness. The names, information, and some of the details of those described have been changed to protect confidentiality. Some of the areas I find my clients often struggle with include:

1. General wellness

2. Weight management

3. Chronic illness or pain

4. Life-balance issues

5. Mood or motivation concerns

6. Relationship struggles

7. Career and finance concerns

8. Trauma

9. Spirituality concerns

10. Addictions

As I share a few case studies these areas, I'm hopeful that you'll be able to see some patterns that will help you as you make important changes in your own life. If your struggles are more severe, work with a trusted therapist to find solutions that will help you.

COMMON WELLNESS CHALLENGES: STORIES FROM THE TRENCHES

Weight Management

Jane's story: "I'm sick of diets. I hate my body."

I think Jane looked at me like most weight management patients do: *Here we go again. Another guy telling me to eat differently, work out harder, and stop being a failure.* Very quickly, I discovered that Jane was burned out. "I just can't do this anymore. I have tried to get up at 5:00 a.m. again and again; I have tried to eat more vegetables and cut out snacks; I have tried to look good for my husband. I just don't seem able to do it. I hate my body. I hate me." It was almost like a confession.

As I do with most clients, I asked Jane to pretend weight was not a problem and that she wasn't there for her weight. I asked, "How are you doing?" She started to talk about her weight again, but I interrupted and said, "No, not your weight. You are not your weight. How are *you* doing?"

She stared at me blankly and then looked away. She started to cry. "I feel beaten down. I feel alone. I don't know. I don't think I'm doing very well."

I listened to Jane's story as she described her relationship with her husband as distant and cold. She described her role as a mother. She felt guilty about snapping at her kids and not keeping up on their homework needs. She felt tired, guilty, and depressed.

After listening to Jane and the heavy burdens that were weighing on her soul, I said, "Life has been hard lately. Sounds like there are some important pieces in your life that aren't quite where you would like them to be." I asked Jane about her years as a teenager. "When you were young, what did you want out of life? What were your dreams? What did you imagine your life to be like?"

She began to reminisce and said, "I guess I wanted what everyone wants—a loving husband, great kids, the house and picket fence . . . the whole thing. You know, the American dream."

"Let me ask you in a different way. When you were a teen, when were you the happiest? What were you doing or who were you with?" Jane began to think and a lightbulb went on. "I loved to sing. I was in a choir and loved to connect with the music. I actually started to write music and play the piano and sing. I really enjoyed it."

"Are you involved in music today?" I asked.

"No, I am not. I mean, I sing at church, but that's about it."

I asked Jane to consider how her life would be today if things were in a place that she could find more joy and peace with herself and others. We brainstormed together. It seemed really important to her to find peace in her soul through music. We began to work on some goals to help her start playing and singing more. She was a little confused, but I explained, "Weight is connected to your life. It is important to have a well life in order to have a well body. This seems important to your life."

When Jane had originally filled out her Life Integration Wheel, I noticed that she was low in love and intimacy and in family and friendships, and she had placed a question mark on life purpose. She was highest in learning because she enjoyed reading a lot and watching documentaries. I connected that desire to learn with music and developed some goals to spend time every day to sing, write music, or play. She came back the next week and said she had enjoyed her week very much, especially the time she spent playing the piano. She mentioned that her youngest kids didn't even know she really liked music. They sat next to her and enjoyed listening to her play. I asked her if she would like to help her kids learn to love music like she did. We decided she would continue to spend time finding ways to include more music in her life the next week and also spend some time sharing this talent with her kids.

The following week, she came back and described how much better her energy level was and how she and her younger kids were getting along better. We discussed the new connection she had made: Doing something she loves while sharing her talents with kids was helping her to have a stronger relationship with them. She felt closer to them.

The next week, she mentioned that she and her husband had engaged in intimacy for the first time in a long time. She said her husband had mentioned he noticed a new spark in her eyes. He said he had missed her and wanted to be closer to her. They began spending more time together.

The following week, she mentioned she had started to look at her life differently. I reminded her she had placed a question mark on her life purpose section of the wheel. She said she had been thinking about this and had come to realize that her music was a way to connect with others, love them, and support them. "I think part of my life purpose is to reach others. I am starting to do this with music. It's helping me connect with both my children and my husband.

She then asked, "Wasn't I coming here to lose weight?"

"Is that still important to you? Why would you want to think about that?" I asked.

"I think what I am realizing is that sometimes my body gets in the way of who I am and what I want to do," she considered. We discussed some of these thoughts and came to the conclusion that really what was impacting her was her energy level. She mentioned she got tired at times, which got in the way of enjoying her day with herself and her family.

"Well, maybe we should focus on energy next? What gets in the way of your energy?" I asked. We came to the conclusion together that when she was up and about she had more energy. She also noticed that she felt better when she drank water instead of Diet Coke. We decided to make a goal of doing something active that she enjoys each day and to start drinking water instead of other drinks. In the end, after some brainstorming, she used some time in the morning to walk around the neighborhood and listen to music while she walked. She used this time to think, meditate, and create melodies in her head. She really looked forward to this each day. She started to invite some friends during some days as well, which added to the enjoyment.

Fast-forward a couple of months, and Jane had actually lost about twenty pounds. More important, she was much happier. She was more connected to her family and husband. She enjoyed life more.

So what happened? I really never talked about weight. Why was she able to lose a significant amount of weight over a year's time without discussing weight that much?

The important principle to learn here is that her weight was a symptom of much deeper pain. Jane's weight concerns were connected to her loneliness, relationships, depression, lack of direction or purpose, and loss of personal passions. Jane had been on so many diets and programs that she knew how to eat and exercise, but she didn't know how to tap into the natural gifts she already had and use those gifts to connect with the world more fully. Once she was connected more to her husband and family, her thoughts and emotions began to change. Serotonin was naturally released in her brain, which acted like a natural antidepressant. Motivation to stay connected and engage in what she loves through her music increased, which acted as a natural support system and long-term motivator. Desire to have the energy to live life was strengthened, which led to a desire to eat better and engage in more physical activity. Her love for music and her family helped heal her. The healing led to a desire to help heal others. Healing others led to a desire to have more energy to be able to heal. The vehicle to lose weight was already there. She knew what to do. We needed to put gas in the vehicle, which ended up being service, relationships and music.

The key to Jane's weight management in this case was through her relationships and passion for music. Spending time and energy on those key aspects of her life is what actually helped her manage her weight. What a mistake it would have been if I had focused on healthy eating and fitness alone. Now, Jane is not just managing her weight, she is managing her life.

In general, I have noticed the following with those struggling with weight management:

Motivation. This is the key; you have to find your true motivation and align your life with it. The rest will come.

Relationships. I have noticed most people addressing weight are really addressing pain. Many need to heal with a spouse, family, higher power, and themselves. Once healed or on track to heal, natural support is created to feel accepted and feel valued. People struggling with weight often feel judged and devalued. Relationship connection trumps devaluation.

Mental and Emotional Health. Thoughts and emotions take time to change but seem to change quicker through relationship healing and tapping into those natural motivations. In Jane's case, her self-defeating thoughts and depression were never directly addressed. Rather, we replaced them by having her engage in activities that naturally changed her thoughts and emotions through relationship building and enjoying music. The most beautiful comment I received from Jane was, "I love me. All of me."

Physicality. When motivation, relationships, thoughts, and emotions are in order, the fitness and nutrition changes become a natural fit. The good vibes we have inside ourselves attract good behaviors for our body. Most know what to do in this area. It is more a matter of using our physical body to meet our most human, sincere desires and needs.

Spirituality. Weight management is often connected to deep spiritual pain. Most people don't want to go there. Our self-esteem or how we value ourselves is often connected to how we believe others value us, including God or a higher power. Once we accept, forgive, and value ourselves through these changes, we often connect deeper with our higher power.

Other areas. It is not uncommon for some individuals to engage in addictive behaviors or activities that replace important life experiences they could be having. These include things like overwork, spending too much money, or engaging in impulses like gambling or pornography. It is important to realize that most of these life balance and addictive issues have their genesis because the individual is in emotional pain. Once the person heals pain and learns to replace these behaviors with long-term healing activities, these areas seem to go away.

In summary, consider all the factors that influence your life as you consider weight. Most of the time, weight is not about weight. Most of the time, spending time on other areas besides our weight will actually make the most difference.

Chronic Pain and Illness

Gary's story: "I'm in pain all the time"

When I first met Gary, I could tell he was in pain. He had suffered through multiple back and hip surgeries and was on high doses of pain medications. I was asked to meet with Gary because his physicians were at a point where they couldn't prescribe any more medications for his pain. Gary's main goal for our meeting was to convince me to tell the physicians to prescribe him more medications. That was his sole focus.

We started out with some small talk. I asked him where he was from and what he used to do before he had become disabled. Originally from Georgia, he described being actively involved in a local Baptist church but had eventually left after a divorce with his wife and what he called a "falling out" with God.

"God and I don't talk anymore. We don't see eye to eye," he said. I learned that he was angry with God because he felt abandoned. He felt everyone had abandoned him, including God.

"It sounds like you have more than just physical pain." I observed. He looked at me blankly and then looked off into the distance out the window. After a while, he said, "Yes, I'm in a lot of pain. I just want it to go away."

That conversation began our journey of discovery as he began to release some of the pain by talking about his ex-wife, friends who became distant after he lost his health, his inability to play football or go cycling due to his back pain, and, eventually, his fall out with God. Some pain gets released when someone feels understood. It is like a too-full balloon that needs some of the air to come out. Telling someone about the pain does not get rid of it all, but it does reduce it.

I asked Gary if he had told anyone about his pain besides me. "Of course. I tell the doctors every month," he said.

"No, not that pain. The other pains," I explained.

He said he did have a girlfriend but that she wouldn't fully understand. "She gets sick of me being in pain all the time, I don't want to burden her with other worries," Gary asserted.

I asked Gary if he would be willing to tell his girlfriend, Sherry, about some of the emotional pain he felt. He agreed, and we decided to meet again.

The following week, Gary came in and was heavily medicated. He was having a hard time paying attention and staying awake. He was able to tell me that he felt closer to his girlfriend this week because they were able to have some serious talks about his past, including some of his previous life. I told him I would like to meet her and invited both of them to the next meeting.

I was surprised when I met Sherry. She was bubbly, positive, and seemed to adore Gary. After some small talk, I learned that Sherry had experienced her own hardships in life following an abusive relationship with an ex-husband. She felt Gary was so kind, and they did have a common interest in being in nature. Sherry was happy to be with Gary. In our meeting, she expressed a desire to help with his pain and allow herself to enter into Gary's world more. Gary was able to say, "I feel like I'm always a burden. I don't want you to worry or listen to my complaining."

Sherry, a little bothered, said, "That's what we do when we love one another. When you don't share with me, I feel you may not want me to be a part of your life. You might not want me."

Gary was a little dumbfounded. "Of course I want you around. I thought if I shared those things, you would go away. When I shared my pain in the past, my wife left me and I lost my job. I don't want to lose anything else." There was a great understanding in this conversation. Once Gary and Sherry began opening up more to one another, I was able to allow Sherry to replace me in my role as listener. Sherry was able to be the person in Gary's life who could listen to his pains and try to understand them. She could be available when I could not. This step opened the door to a complete shift in Gary's life and wellness.

Although this took some time, the first piece of the puzzle fell into place when I we noticed how Gary had scored himself on his Life Integration Wheel. His "play and fun" were really down because he couldn't engage in some of the sports he used to play. He was also low in love and intimacy, spirituality, and the professional sphere. After the breakthrough with Sherry, his love and intimacy had skyrocketed, but the "play and fun" area also began to increase as Gary and Sherry started visiting national parks and other nature areas. Although they couldn't engage in long, strenuous hikes, Gary was able to engage in some short hikes over time, especially when he enjoyed the area and was with Sherry. The increase in physical activity coupled with a relationship that allowed him to confide in someone helped to decrease in depression. Engaging in hobbies he enjoyed started to reduce his pain. As his mood changed, he naturally started to change his diet and also spent more time reading and learning new skills like woodworking.

Those who suffer from chronic pain or illness know that sometimes just sitting there thinking about the pain can drive you nuts. When Gary was learning, reading, or doing something he enjoyed, his mind was elsewhere. In many ways, he was practicing mindfulness as he stayed in the present enjoying the activity at hand.

The final piece of Gary's puzzle was his relationship with God. He finally told me one day, "I'm starting to talk to God again. We still don't see eye to eye, but I am starting to feel that maybe He didn't abandon me." Gary's healing process with his spirituality was slow, but in the end he found peace in volunteering at a local church and working with the youth again. His "professional" part of the wheel increased along with "life purpose" as he discovered a need to help others come to peace with life amidst all the hardships life gives.

In the end, we did not need to increase his pain medications. Rather, we increased his connection with his girlfriend and others, his time spent in enjoying nature and learning hobbies that didn't increase his pain, and his healing with his past and with God. The key to Gary's wellness plan was helping him realize there is much life to live beyond the pain and that much of that life can help alleviate that pain.

One of my favorite moments with Gary was when he said, "I never thought my life after my accident could be this happy. I can't believe I almost let physical pain take away peace and love in my life."

In general, I have noticed the following with those struggling with chronic pain or even chronic illness:

Emotional and Mental Health. I have noticed that many people dealing with physical pain have forgotten about their emotional pain, either from the past or in the present. They focus so much on the physical that their emotional side becomes "infected." Helping people address their emotional pain actually helps them reduce their physical pain and change their mood and attitude toward life. Healing emotional pain actually heals some of the physical pain. It also seems to change the way chronic sufferers think about life.

Physicality. Actively engaging in some type of cardio, especially outside, seems to help reduce pain and increase mood. I usually try to tie the physical to an activity the client truly enjoys or something that offers them the opportunity to spend more time with loved ones.

Motivation. As people heal and start thinking about the present and future, aligning someone's life with their true passions, interests, and life purpose is important for someone with pain or illness. It is not uncommon for people in pain or illness to identify themselves as the illness or ailment. Instead, they need to identify themselves as someone with much to offer others and much to learn and experience with life.

Relationships. Many people with pain or illness feel like a burden on others. They also feel misunderstood. It is important to help someone in pain or illness connect and not distance. I have also found it beneficial to introduce new people in their life through support groups or associations in which others are experiencing similar things.

Spirituality. Pain is often connected to spirituality, because many find peace and healing through a higher power. For others, spirituality adds to a deeper sense of meaning and purpose for their life.

Other areas. It is not uncommon for those dealing with pain to want to numb the pain through more medication or even drugs, sex, alcohol, and other impulsive behaviors. The key here is helping people learn to heal pain through other means.

In summary, consider all the factors that influence your life as you consider pain or illness. Most of the time, the key is stepping back and realizing your life doesn't have to only be about pain or an illness. Most of the time, focusing on therapeutic options other than medication management will actually make the most difference.

Depression and Anxiety
Susanne's story: "I'm burned out on life."

I never worked with Susanne personally. But she described her experience to me as a professional colleague. Susanne was working as an executive in a firm in downtown Chicago. She was a working mother with two young children and a husband who was a physician. Although she was successful in her career, she was feeling burned out on life. "I just don't feel motivated to get

up and go to work every day. I enjoy what I do at work, and I enjoy my colleagues, but there is something missing in my life, and I'm afraid I will wake
up ten years from now and not know who I even am anymore," she would say.
As I talked with Susanne off and on, it was really important to her to be true
to herself. She began to realize that the amount of time and energy she was
spending on her career was taking away time from some of her other dreams
and goals in life.

In addition, because she was feeling out of alignment, she noticed her relationship with her kids and husband were off. There was a general feel of stress
and distance at home. She also mentioned letting herself go physically because
she didn't have energy or time to go to the local yoga studio or eat consistently
like she used to. Instead, she would skip meals or grab something quick that
really didn't fit her food wants. She also noticed that she was not getting the
rest she needed when she slept.

Over time, Susanne discovered that she felt she was missing some elements
in her life that were important to her. As we discussed her options, Susanne
always talked about her time in the Peace Corps in South America. She loved
helping the communities and giving service. She knew that the happiness she
felt then was missing from her life now and wanted to get that sense of having
an impact for good back into her life. At one point, she was so gung-ho about
getting back into nonprofit work that she made the decision to quit her job and
start her own nonprofit. "This is going to take a lot of energy and time—two
commodities you are already low on," I reminded her. She agreed, and after
thinking about the problem some more, Susannne eventually negotiated with
her current employer to work reduce her work hours from forty per week to
thirty hours per week. She also requested to have Fridays off and to have the
option to telecommute from home on two of the remaining days each week. By
reducing her work hours this way, she also saved commuting time. Her weekly
work obligations reduced from sixty-five hours per week to thirty.

Susanne was excited about the change. In reality, the amount of money
she would be earning was not that much less, and her husband still received
health insurance and other benefits from his work, so her financial wellness
safety net was still in place. The first things Susanne put back into her daily
routine were yoga and cooking meals at home (another love she had lost over
the years). She also was able to take her kids to school and see them when they
got home. The main purpose for her change though was to get more involved
in service. She was excited to join a local nonprofit that worked hand in hand
with the Peace Corps in South America. She gave this organization about
twenty hours of her time per month, with an annual trip. She looked forward

to the day when her kids would be old enough to be involved with the group in the future as well.

As the changes she made began to settle, the relationship with her husband and kids improved, her health and energy improved drastically, and her love for life was rekindled with a restructuring of how she spent her time. As an added bonus, the vice president of the company told her she was actually doing better work now that she was working only thirty hours a week than she had been when she had been spending longer hours. The key to Susanne's changes was a desire to be true to herself. In other words, she wanted to align her life (time, roles, and responsibilities) to what was important to her rather than let life rule her.

In this example, it's important to note that Susanne was able to make these changes on her own *without* the help of professionals. Technically, Susanne had enough symptoms to be diagnosed with depression. Even though counseling and medications could have helped her on some level, the restructuring and balancing of her life tapped into the natural serotonin of her body and improved her support system. In addition, the exercise and eating added to the needed energy and boosted her mood as well. Susanne told me later on, "I love my life."

In general, I have noticed the following with those struggling with feeling down or depressed:

Life Balance. For many with depression, the symptoms come from a lack of serotonin in the brain. Although some of this is genetic, it is common for low serotonin to stem from stress, distant relationships, poor health, and lack of direction in life. Addressing the roles and how we spend our time can often improve our mood and energy because we are able to devote more time and energy to areas that improve our emotional, mental, relational, and physical well-being.

Emotions and Thoughts. When working with someone who is depressed, it is common for a therapist to help a client change their thought processes and behaviors to impact their emotions. I have found that many of those thoughts and behaviors will change as a client finds their true life purpose and restructures their life to include behaviors like hobbies, family, spirituality, and exercise in a way that will provide a natural serotonin boost.

Physicality. Cardio is important for those dealing with depression or anxiety. Engaging in cardio that you enjoy is even more important.

Relationships. Because many people distance themselves or get irritable with people when experiencing depression, it is common for people with depression to isolate themselves or push people away. Reconnecting and healing relationships has been shown to alleviate many depressive symptoms.

Motivation. When someone has depression, they are not motivated. Sometimes people need to just start engaging in activity they know they will like or learn to like even if they don't feel like it. You have to get over that hump. Having faith that your motivation will return is key.

Spirituality. Similar to pain, those with depression often find spirituality to be a healing balm to their symptoms.

Other areas. Some people with depression try to engage in behaviors that help them sleep more or forget their pain. Some will use sleeping pills, over-medicate, or engage in "downers" to help them sleep away their lives. It is not uncommon for people to learn different ways to heal and relax as they learn to cope with pain differently.

In summary, consider all the factors that influence your life as you consider depression. I do recommend a counselor and some medication at times when it can jump-start the process. However, most success seems to come from the other elements in our life that help us be happy.

Trauma

Hank's story: "I can't stop thinking about it. I relive it every day."

Trauma is difficult. Hank had been back from Afghanistan for about nine months. He was a young father with three kids ranging from six years old to nine months old. He came to my office with what we call a "flat affect." In other words, no expression on his face—no affect. He had bags under his eyes, was skinny and long, and wore clothes that were dirty and smelled of grease. "Hey, Doc," he said politely. I got to know Hank a little bit that day. He had been through several tours, with his last tour being difficult because he lost a number of friends in combat. His wife had asked him to come see me because she was worried that "he was not himself."

I asked Hank how he was doing, and he said, "Oh, things are fine. You know getting back into the swing of things . . ." He trailed off and looked off in the distance. "Oh, sorry, Doc. My mind wanders a bit sometimes."

"Where does it wonder to?" I asked. "Oh, you know, just things . . ." and he trailed off again. I could imagine how his wife must feel. Hank wasn't fully present; he was somewhere else. I'm sure his children wondered why their dad wasn't fully there as well. We decided to meet again next week. I think he liked getting out of the house because he didn't want to listen to his wife yell at him again for this or that.

The following week, Hank was the same—distant, polite, and not fully present. Because Hank was not allowing me in, I knew this would be a slow process. Trauma sufferers often create barriers to protect themselves and others from facing immense pain. When they face this pain, they feel out of control and are fearful of doing something they will regret. Rather than focus on the trauma he was obviously experiencing, I thought I would get to know him more. I discovered he loved his dog Charlie. "Tell me about Charlie," I asked.

"Charlie is a great dog. He is always there for me and expects nothing from me. He loves me no matter what," he said. I learned from that brief statement that he may be wondering if others love him because he is not meeting their expectations. I asked if I could meet Charlie.

Hank had mentioned that he enjoyed skipping rocks out by a local lake, so we spent the following meeting playing with his dog and skipping rocks. It was a peaceful place. "I come here to forget," Hank said. I didn't want to push, so I said nothing. He quietly said, "You see, I can't stop thinking about it. I relive it every day." It turns out that Hank was thinking a lot about an experience he had in Afghanistan when a good friend died. I learned that day that Hank was stuck. He said, "I don't know what to do. I don't want to forget him, but when I think about him, I panic. I'm taken back to that place."

"I wonder if there would be a way to remember him and honor him but not have to panic?" I pondered out loud with him.

"That's what I would want," he said sadly, thinking it wouldn't likely ever happen.

The brain is a marvelous thing. We know that thoughts are associated with experiences and memories through pathways. These pathways can be rebuilt to associate a thought or memory to different emotions and experiences. The pathways associated with trauma are usually pretty ingrained because that person usually thinks about it often and it is associated with fear or danger. The key to helping Hank would be to help him associate his friend with different emotions and experiences. In addition, you can't ever do this alone. He had Charlie, and he was beginning to trust me, but he needed others in his life. I asked if I could meet his wife alone. He agreed.

Jill was a great woman. She was kind and adored Hank. She missed him a lot. She was also overwhelmed taking care of the bills, family, household, and so on. "I don't know what to do," she said. "I know he is hurting, but he won't talk to me. I feel helpless," she said as she teared up. This was a family in a lot of pain.

This took quite a bit of time, but we ended up having meetings with Hank and slowly brought Jill into some of the meetings. She learned how to help

Hank release some of the pain as the anxiety came and how to stop when it was going too far. At the same time, individual counseling sessions with Hank gave me the opportunity to help him release as well. It is important to note that when we refer to "releasing pain," the release involves the person sharing memories and feelings associated with the pain. It is important to be under the guidance of a trained professional for this process. Eventually, enough of Hank's pain and traumatic experiences had been released that he began to look in the present more, and then we brought his family to the meetings. This was a wonderful step as his children began to play more with him and he played with them.

As Hank became more present, some of his health concerns began to turn around. He ate more consistently and didn't throw up as much in the mornings due to his anxiety. He also started to run in the mornings with Charlie, which increased his serotonin and improved his mood. He was drinking a lot of energy drinks while working on base to stay awake because he wasn't sleeping well. As he exercised and ate better, he was able to sleep better and eventually gave up the energy drinks for the most part. Slowly, Hank and his wife were able to form a much deeper connection. The trauma became a vehicle that solidified their relationship. They became 100-percent loyal to each other, and the fear of not meeting expectations or someone leaving the relationship was gone. Hank also started to attend church with his family and eventually began coaching baseball for his son with some of the other boys at church. His isolation turned into connection with others in his community.

The principles of WholeFIT in this situation played out by helping Hank with his thoughts and emotions first, while slowly introducing family and friends to his life for support. His physical health easily fell into place once he was on track to let go of some of the pain and connect with others. His life purpose shifted as he was more present with his family. In the end, family became his life, and everything else pointed to that.

At one point in our journey, Hank said, "You know, I still think about Jim, and it is painful, but it doesn't get in the way anymore. It actually motivates me to never take the life I have for granted. I want to spend time on what is important to me. At this point, family is my everything."

In general, I have noticed the following with those struggling with trauma:

Emotions and Thoughts. Those who are dealing with trauma have challenges related to the thoughts and emotions associated with the trauma. A trained professional familiar with trauma is highly recommended because this can be a delicate process. In general, most people need a slow release of the pain by talking through the trauma gradually, while reintroducing their life to areas that will improve thoughts and mood, like family, hobbies, and spirituality.

Relationships. It is common for those dealing with trauma to isolate themselves. Family members and friends need to be aware of how to connect with someone dealing with trauma and recognize patience will be needed. A professional can help guide this process. In the end, most will find a lot of healing through their relationships.

Physicality. When trauma is present, the body reacts physically. Difficulty eating and sleeping is common, while some will overeat or throw up when anxiety is present. Others may engage in addictive substances to numb the pain. Equally, the body will often experience physical pain and tightness. Cardio, weight lifting, and eating healthily usually comes as the person heals the pain. Once a person is far enough along in the healing process, engaging in physical activity and healthy eating becomes much easier.

Spirituality. Similar to pain and depression, spirituality can provide a great social and healing resource. Some have found prayer or meditation to be helpful as the person releases some of these thoughts.

Motivation. One thing I have noticed with trauma is that once people heal enough, they are likely to have a much easier time than most in finding what is most important to them. I think what happens is that the trauma somehow washes away all the unnecessary worries of life and allows them to focus more, with many dedicating their life to family, service, and spirituality.

Life Balance. Because trauma impacts all areas of life, finding balance in all areas will greatly improve someone's chance to heal. It is a slow process, but trying to do small things in each of the areas of our lives can help.

Other areas. Helping others seems to be helpful for people struggling with trauma. Also, being in nature, being around animals, or serving others can be healing. Music, the arts, and hobbies are also helpful because they distract the mind and provide some peace for a moment.

In summary, consider all the factors that influence your life as you consider dealing with trauma. I do recommend a professional counselor and a great support system. Trauma impacts all areas of our lives, and all areas impact trauma. A wholistic approach is likely to bring healing quicker.

Intimacy

Lila's story: "I don't know my husband anymore. I feel alone."

Lila related her experience to me and my wife as mutual friends. Although

Lila and her husband had been to marriage counseling off and on for years, they still struggled. Like many couples, they felt distant from one another and overworked—both at home and on the job. They had three children, and both of them worked. They had been married for twelve years. Steve had gained some weight over the years, partially from working too much and partially from emotionally eating away his stress. Lila and Steve struggled with intimacy and considered themselves more like roommates or even business partners. They were on a consistent schedule to make everything work but didn't really fight or spend much time together. At one point, Lila related, "I don't know my husband anymore. We are like strangers. I looked at him the other day and realized, *I don't know this man and he doesn't know me*. I feel alone." From my experience, I knew this was the perfect formula for an affair. I hoped that wouldn't happen because it can be so difficult to heal from something like that.

I didn't see Lila for a couple of months and then ran into her at the grocery store. I asked how things were going. She looked different. "It's amazing what has happened. I'm a different person," she radiated.

"Wow, what happened?" I asked, wondering if she was going to tell me she met some handsome guy, got divorced, and is now living in a bed-and-breakfast or something.

"You know, I can't fully explain it, but it started with holding hands," she shared. "We were sitting on the couch, and Steve held my hand."

After talking with her for a little bit in the grocery store, I forgot about our conversation and didn't see her again for another couple of months. I ran into her at the store again. This time, Lila was glowing. Last time she was happy, but now she seemed to have a hop in her step.

"Hey, how's it going?" I asked.

"Life is good, Jared. Things are good," she smiled. Eventually, I found out what happened. From my own perspective, I think what occurred is that when Lila and Steve held hands that night, they had reached a tipping point. They were about to make a decision to keep distancing and say good-bye emotionally or to start again. They chose to start again amidst all the fear, stress, and loneliness. They started small by sitting by each other each night and holding hands. They began to talk to each other between shows or during the commercials and eventually would turn the TV off completely. Conversation started with things about kids, school, or work. Then they started to talk about their future—hopes, dreams, and desires. As they learned more about each other, they started to invite each other to do things together they enjoyed. Lila enjoyed walking in the evenings and invited Steve along. They started cooking together at night, and the kids joined in. The intimacy and energy that came from exercising together and spending time together led to a natural inclination to eat better and relax more. They started to vacation more. They started to engage in more hobbies like photography and painting, and they shared in each other's hobbies. The kids paid attention to the changes and started to spend more time on outdoor activities and hobbies rather than Netflix and iPhones. Both Lila and Steve also adjusted how they spent their time in the evenings and at work. Work was not the main focus anymore; it was a means to an end. They set boundaries on themselves and said no a lot more and yes to more of the right things.

In Lila's situation, it was clear that the WholeFIT principles that were most important in this situation were starting with the marital relationship. As they got to know each other again, their love and connection shifted their thinking, hopes, and life direction. How they spent time on work, where they placed importance on family and hobbies, how they impacted their kids, and how they treated their bodies all stemmed from the connection they created with each other. Sometimes, our bodies, minds, and lives will be most impacted through the healing of a relationship.

It is interesting that each of the people in the previous stories who needed a change started by going through a different door. For some, the door to wellness is thoughts, for others it is a relationship, and for others it is spirituality. However, each door eventually leads to changes in all areas. Lila told me once, "I was ready to accept the fact that my life with Steve would be like this forever. I realize now through small, simple changes how whole lives can shift dramatically. We are in love, and we love life."

In general, I have noticed the following with those struggling with a marital relationship:

Emotions and Thoughts. Experience has shown me the importance of tapping into the emotional side of our relationship. There is usually fear here—fear of loss or rejection or apathy. Sometimes this emotion is accessed through touch, like Lila explained, or through conversation or spending time together. Once these emotions of wanting to be together and care for one another are released and accepted, the love begins to grow. Our thoughts change, our behaviors change, and the way we view life changes.

Motivation. I've noticed that when couples begin to align themselves and connect with one another, having the couple talk about their motivations, passions, life purpose, and life direction can shift their thinking to the present and future rather than the pains of the past. The couple gets excited, and they start to engage in life and planning more together.

Physicality. For many couples, finding a way to *connect* is the catalyst to change, and connecting emotionally tends to give them more opportunities to exercise and eat well—together. For others, it works the other way around. Changing their fitness and nutrition patterns so that they eat together and exercise more increases the intimacy.

Spirituality. It is not uncommon for intimacy to melt into spirituality because they often come from the same cloth. In other words, couples will naturally have spiritual conversations and engage in spiritual practices as their intimacy increase. Spiritual activities like meditation, attending religious meetings, or praying or reading together from spiritual material (scripture, or inspirational readings) sometimes increases when their intimacy increases because spirituality shared with others is intimate.

Life Balance. As the couple connects, the connection bleeds over to family. Their views of life changes as their relationships become the focus for their happiness. Life naturally begins to be restructured to support the intimacy.

In summary, consider all the factors that influence your life as you work on your relationships. It is common to focus on the relationship itself. Remember, the relationship is only one piece of the puzzle. When we consider working on our relationship within the context of our whole life with all the pieces at hand, we are more likely to make changes that last because now our whole life reflects the intimacy of our relationships.

Addictions

Phil's story: "My addiction is killing me."

When I first met Phil, he was a successful surgeon with a wife and two young kids. I didn't know he was hiding an addiction. No one really knew about his addiction. His life had started to unravel, and it wasn't clear what was going on to most people. I eventually had a frank talk with him. "What are you using?" I asked.

"What do you mean?" he said, dumbfounded.

"Listen, I'm not trying to hurt you or embarrass you or anything, but I want to help you before something serious happens. We need to make a shift now, or things will start to slide quickly," I said.

Phil looked at me a long time. "Heroine," he whispered. "I started with pain pills and medications, and now it is heroine." Phil and I started making a plan, but I soon realized I was making the plan and he was only nodding. I was in crisis mode, and he was chill. I was working harder than he was. I found out that he felt he could maintain his life with his addiction. He didn't want to change.

I didn't hear from Phil or his family for three weeks. His wife finally called me and asked to come in.

"We are getting a divorce. Phil was tested at work, and he has been fired from the hospital. He will likely lose his medical license because he was stealing drugs and money from the hospital for a long time," she said as she cried.

This story is sad. Phil lost his job, his license, and his family. His wife eventually found a boyfriend who became abusive. The kids were scarred, traumatized, and hurting for years. Phil eventually went to treatment and became a lab technician after becoming sober for a period. He relapsed a couple of times. I met Phil again two years later. "My addiction is killing me. Not just my body, it is killing my life. My wife hates me, my ex-wife hates me, my kids don't trust me, and I don't trust me. Jared, I need help for real. I'm lost," he sobbed.

It is common for people in addiction to have to hit rock bottom to really move forward. "Okay, let's begin," I said. As the twelve-steps program suggests, the first step is recognizing our lives have become unmanageable. Phil went through many ups and downs, but the key for Phil was starting with loving and forgiving himself. He had come from a family with very high expectations. He tied his self-esteem and self-identity to achievement. If he failed, he was unlovable. If he succeeded, he was lovable. We had to do significant work with him forgiving his father, letting go of the high expectations of his mother, and, eventually, learning to see himself as someone who could be loved in spite of making mistakes. At the same time, we needed something to give him drive and not cross-addict. Cross-addiction happens when someone replaces one addiction with another to continue to numb the pain. As Phil began to forgive and love himself, he replaced his addiction with running. Running moved to cycling and swimming, and eventually he became a very competitive triathlon athlete. He began to reach out to his ex-wife and children and ask for forgiveness with no expectation of a return. They were hesitant. His daughter still has not forgiven him; she is not ready. But Phil is okay with that, knowing that he can only do his part. He and his son, by contrast, have a good relationship.

Phil has been clean for seven years. His body has changed, his mind has changed, and his view on life has changed. He is a spiritual person but not a religious person. Most important, he defines himself differently. Phil told me once, "I once saw myself as a surgeon or an important person in the community. My value was tied to how others saw me, but I was empty inside. I had nothing to offer others really. I understand where my relationship failed. I thought what she wanted was a position, a status, and an income. She wanted love, and my kids wanted love, and I didn't have it to give because I didn't even have it for myself. I now have love, and I can give that to others. Drugs numbed my emptiness but only added to it. I now can love. I hope I can always love."

In the end, the key to Phil's success was to focus on how he valued himself. If he were to fill out a Life Integration Wheel, the key areas that I would have focused on would be his self-esteem and life purpose areas. Because those areas were really a facade, his whole life became a facade. As he learned how to value himself and understand how to align that value with life, he could then begin to fill the emptiness and heal his pain. He could now offer something to others that was tangible—love. Relationships could be formed and developed for the first time, and how he treated his body and spirit became a shadow of how he treated himself. Phil now has many chapters in his book of life to write, and he is hopeful.

In general, I have noticed the following with those struggling with an addiction:

Self-Esteem and Life Purpose. I have noticed that many with addiction are trying to numb pain or fill a void. This is often tied to how they view themselves and how they think others value them. Learning to love and forgive yourself and discover your life purpose based on real values is important when addressing addictions.

Relationships. It is common for the values and identity of an addict to stem from relationships that have left wounds. Sometimes, parents, partners, or friends have left an impression on us that communicates a certain value. As we heal these relationships or memories and learn to offer others true value and our true self, we begin to connect with others. As we seek forgiveness, we can let go of the past.

Emotions and Thoughts. Addicts' brains change when using. They actually replace memories, emotions, and experiences with the feeling of the drug. As an addict changes, emotions and thoughts return. This can be difficult because these emotions and thoughts are often painful. When pain returns, it is important to find different ways to heal this pain, and often that doesn't happen without first improving relationships, developing spirituality, and finding life purpose. As we change, our thoughts and emotions change. For most, it takes at least a year.

Motivation. When the addiction or maintaining the addiction is no longer the goal, life becomes full of possibilities. Aligning our life purpose with motivation is important. Most addicts replace the drug with a motivation to serve, learn, and grow.

Physicality. Just as the mind changes, the body also changes due to addiction. Some addictions cause us to become physically dependent, while others cause psychological dependency. In other words, our bodies require that we have this addiction in our lives to feel normal. As the addict changes, the body changes. It will be painful. Fitness and nutrition can help speed up the process.

Spirituality. The twelve-step program and other programs addressing addiction tap into spirituality because it is common for someone with an addiction to need to find forgiveness and meaning from a higher power. The greatest desire for many is to find peace. Peace with ourselves, peace with others, and peace with God.

Life Balance. Similar to trauma, those who have experienced addiction have experienced a self-inflicted trauma. Thus, life balance seems to come easier to someone who has healed from an addiction because they realize what is truly important. They structure their lives to give themselves time and energy for what is most important to them, which often involves family, serving others, and connecting with a higher power.

In summary, consider all the factors that influence your life as you work through an addiction. An addiction is pervasive. It impacts all areas of our life. It becomes clear that a long-term approach to healing an addiction must include all these areas. Many will relapse over and over again. The people I have noticed that have truly become clean make a significant shift in how they view themselves, others, and life.

CONCLUSION

Each story shared in this chapter has a common thread: All areas of health and wellness are connected, and improving in one of these areas creates a domino effect on the others. When we consider our own health and wellness, we can't just think about what we eat or how we lift weights. Health and wellness means aligning our true self with what is most important to us. Our healthy and well self includes our relationships, life purpose, motivations, passions, career, thoughts, emotions, and spirituality. When we realize all of these areas are connected, we begin to find the real solutions to our health and wellness.

I wonder if some people might think that a guy writing and compiling a book like this must have this all figured out. I really don't. I have been blessed to learn a lot and gain some experience learning from others. As I said in the beginning, this is some of what we know so far. I am using what I have learned personally to help me have a better life. I continue to struggle to know how to integrate all these areas in my life. That is part of the journey. Some of us are considering getting on the path to wellness, while others are struggling along a path they have already started. I see others and sometimes think they are close to the end of the journey—they have figured it out. Professionally, I'm most worried about the person still deciding to get on the path or not. As long as you are on the path working toward better days, you will move forward. The fact that you are reading this book suggests you are already on the path.

There are a number of stories I thought about sharing in this book based on past clients that are just too difficult for me to share. They are too sacred. I was allowed to witness and participate in people sharing their deepest pains and tragedies with me and watch some of them heal. True healing occurs when we access all that is us—our bodies, minds, hearts, souls, and relationships. It is an amazing experience and has given me a tremendous amount of respect and hope for a human being's ability to overcome. I have also experienced intense sadness and darkness witnessing the tremendous amount of hurt we can give one another and ourselves. None of us are immune from the evils of this world or the harm we can place on ourselves. One thing that gives me hope is thinking of red boots.

Whenever I see a pair of red boots, my mind goes back more than a decade to a little boy that I worked with, who taught me more about resilience, happiness, forgiveness, and hope than anyone before or since. He was five years old—about the same age as my own son is now. This little boy went through horrible, horrible experiences, but he always smiled when he was with me. One day, he received some red boots, and he was so proud. He couldn't contain his excitement when he showed them to me. I have a fond memory ingrained in my mind of watching him walking with his red boots, a huge smile on his face. It is hard to explain why exactly, but for some reason that memory represents to me the chance each of us has for goodness to occur in our lives in spite of all that is placed before us. If he had the ability to walk with a smile after all he went through at such a tender age, I can. We all can. We all can take the steps that move us through the heartache and difficulty and live a better life. A well life.

Many years ago, I was walking along the banks of a sewage river in South America. I remember thinking that it was quite cold that morning as the mud was frozen and I was breaking ice as I stepped in small pockets of water along the trail. I could see my breath. It was early in the morning, and no one was really out. The sun started to peek over the horizon.

I remember seeing a little girl and her younger sister, barefoot, with hardly any clothing on. They were both dragging glass beer bottles across the ground because the full bottles were too heavy to carry. I asked them where they were going. They were wide-eyed and scared—surprised a gringo would be talking to them. They pointed to a shack across the river. I asked to help them, because I could see they were so cold and still needed to cross a dirty, cold river. The younger one, maybe three years old, seemed willing, but the five-year-old rushed them along so they wouldn't be too late getting the alcohol back to their father. They were determined to get his beer to him quickly, despite the harsh conditions.

That experience is also ingrained in my head. I felt such heartache not being able to help. They were so frail and in need. There were thousands like them in the city. I also realized the power this father had. Whether we agree with the task given to the children or not, these children wanted to please their father—maybe out of love, maybe out of fear. What I do know is that some of us can have a greater influence on helping improve an individual's life than others can. We each have a stewardship and responsibility to those whose lives we touch. We have power to help. We also can't do much when we don't have that connection. I realized that day that if I want to help, I need to build trust with that person or I need to access people that have gained trust with them. This is important. As you consider living a well life, find those that you trust and access their help. Equally, help those that have gained your trust. Surround yourself with good people and remove those that harm you in your life.

One final thought: I have learned that many of us fear change. I get it. We know what we are getting from our life now, and sometimes it feels safest to accept our lot in life—even though there may be negative consequences—rather than risk changes. Starting something new or making changes suggests accepting consequences we have not experienced. If I make this change, things may get worse. Things are bad now, but I know I can endure the status quo somehow, while I'm *not* sure I'm equipped to handle things if they get worse.

I have previously mentioned my experience in Houston, where I was a tenure-track professor in a good position at a good school in a wonderful area. However, I was working too much, my health was suffering, and I felt a need to get closer to family. Beyond all reason, I quit my job. I left with no job offer and started anew. It was scary, but I felt I could figure things out with the idea that I would make better decisions this time as I placed higher priorities on my health, family, service, and life enjoyment. Three years later, I am writing this book, healthier than I have been in a long time, closer to my family, less stressed, and making more money than I was in Houston. It worked out. It hasn't always worked out, but it did this time.

Remember, making a change is a risk. I believe that making calculated risks in a way that improves your overall life is worth it in the end. Fear will get in the way at times. Have faith that if you work toward the important things in life, wellness will follow.

I hope we have given you some additional ideas to keep moving forward. In the end, I hope you understand that part of improving wellness is knowing who should be on your team. Your spouse or significant other, family, friends, colleagues, and professionals are all part of your life. One of the goals of the book is to help you consider how all these people can work together more to help you be well.

Equally, part of a wellness plan is knowing how to access good information, good people, and good resources. I hope you can keep finding good people in your community and good information that you need to continue learning how to be well. We don't know everything, and there is much to be discovered. Part of wellness is a desire to keep looking. We are always willing to provide you with additional guidance if needed.

Feel free to contact us at WholeFitWellness.com. I feel we have been on a journey together as you have read and we have shared. I think you know we are sincere in our efforts to help others heal, or to help those who are doing well get even more out of life. I hope you now realize more than before that wellness goes far beyond diets and sit-ups.

We have added an appendix after this chapter to be used as a guide to help develop your own personal wellness plan. It will utilize the principles and concepts introduced in the book to get you started. We also have provided you with a list of several resources that we think can help in the appendix as well. Wellness includes all areas of our life, and that wellness can be for life.

Until next time—happy trails!

APPENDIX

CREATING YOUR PERSONAL WELLNESS PLAN

Step 1: Begin by filling out your own copy of the Life Integration Wheel (see page 11). Make note of any areas where you score particularly high, as well as those where you scored lower.

Step 2: Consider some areas that are going really well in your life, as well as some where you might be struggling.

I'm doing pretty well with _____

_____

_____

And _____

_____

_____

I have an opportunity to improve in these two areas: _____

_____

(Remember "the talk rule" introduced in chapter 2: Talk about what you *do* want more than what you do *not* want).

Step 3: Remember that everything is connected. Are there certain areas in your life or wheel that are connected to your areas of struggle?

Which areas in your life seem to be impacting your struggles the most? _____

_____

_____

_____

How do these areas impact your current struggles? _____

_____

_____

Step 4: After reviewing the case studies from chapter 18, can you identify a different door you might be able to try that would give you a chance to succeed at improving one area of your overall wellness? It may help to ask yourself the following questions:

- If a miracle happened and life was how you would like it to be, what would it look like?

- What drives you?

- What brings you happiness?

- What would be different in your life?

- What would be the same?

- When you were a teen, when were you the happiest? What were you doing or who were you with?

- When was a time in your life or your work that you really experienced "flow?"

Step 5: Answer the question, *"What's getting in the way of having your life look like that?"* _____

_____

_____

The answer to these questions may give you a hint for a different door you can go through as you begin to work on improving your overall wellness. Once you've identified that idea, you may want to start at the beginning with a *different* behavior you are excited about changing. If you are stuck or feel you will not be able to make the needed changes without professional help, make a commitment to seek out the help you need.

Step 6: Next, using the tools you learned in chapter 4, identify an aspect of your personal wellness you think you are ready to take *action* with. (You've passed the preparation stage of change and you are thinking about moving to the action stage.) *Write the one behavior you are considering changing here:* ___

_____

_____

Step 7: Scale the importance of making that change. *On a scale from 0 to 10, where 0 is not important at all and 10 is the most important thing, how important is it for you to [write the behavior you plan to change]?* _____

- What makes it that number?
- Why not a lower number?

Step 8: Now, scale your *confidence* in your ability to make a change:

On a scale from 0 to 10, where 0 is not confident at all and 10 is the most confident, how confident do you feel about being able to [write the behavior you plan to change]? _____

- What makes it that number?
- Why not a lower number?

Step 9: Choose a goal that will help you on your path toward change.

Step 10: Share this goal with your partner or family and consider repeating the steps as a couple or family.

Step 11: Consider writing your goals down and reviewing them often. Reevaluate and tweak your goals over time.

ADDITIONAL RESOURCES

We hope you have enjoyed the principles and ideas portrayed in our book, *WholeFIT: Wellness for Life*. We have received multiple requests to offer readers additional resources for various areas. In addition to the recommended readings, we offer you the following resources:

WholeFIT Coaching and Counseling: We offer health coaching and counseling in Texas, Utah, Arizona, and online. Many of our counselors and coaches are located at various Centers for Couples & Families in each of these states. Locations can be found at Couples-Families.com. In addition, we work in several clinics and wellness centers which can be found at WholeFitWellness.com. Finally, we have an online center that can offer coaching and counseling throughout the country at NetFamilyTherapy.com. We would be happy to help you explore some of these ideas on a more personal level if you feel that would be helpful.

WholeFIT for Medical Clinics, Therapists, and Providers: We currently help a number of clinics and wellness centers integrate behavioral health and wellness into their practices. A special appendix has been written that can be found online at WholeFitWellness.com/special-appendices.html, or visit WholeFitWellness.com to learn more about how WholeFIT can help with collaborative health care, integrative medicine, and patient-centered medicine.

WholeFIT for Corporations and Small Businesses: We currently offer corporate wellness programs to various corporations and small businesses. A special appendix has been written that can be found online addressing WholeFIT for businesses, which can be found at WholeFitWellness.com/special-appendices. html, or visit WholeFitWellness.com to learn more about how WholeFIT can help with productivity, wellness, company culture, and innovation.

Special Appendices Online: As mentioned, we have two additional appendices that can be accessed online at Wholefitwellness.com/special-appendices. html.

- WholeFIT for Medical Providers & Professionals
- WholeFIT for Businesses
- Life Integration Wheel
- Recommended Readings

Custom Fit Workouts: If you would like access to some fitness videos written by the editor to help you get going on your fitness, visit CustomFitWorkouts. com.

Speaking, Training, and Consulting by Dr. Jared DuPree

If you would be interested in having Dr. Jared DuPree speak, train, or consult with you, your group, or your business, contact him at WholeFitWellness. com/contact-us, or visit the Facebook page and other social media sites.

- *Facebook*: facebook.com/wholefitwellness
- *LinkedIn*: linkedin.com/company/wholefit
- *YouTube channel*: youtube.com/c/wholefitwellnessforlife
- *WholeFIT newsletter/blog sign up*: eepurl.com/bxiI2T
- *Twitter*: twitter.com/Whole_FIT
- *Google+*: google.com/+Wholefitwellnessforlife